CATHEDRAL

{ALSO BY BILL HENDERSON}

FICTION

The Kid That Could   Nautilus, 1970

NONFICTION

His Son   Norton, 1981; Quill, 1982

Her Father   Faber and Faber, 1995

Tower: Faith, Vertigo, and Amateur Construction
Farrar, Straus & Giroux, 2000;
North Point Press, 2001

Simple Gifts: One Man's Search for Grace
Free Press, 2006

All My Dogs: A Life   David Godine, 2011

AS EDITOR

The annual *Pushcart Prize* series
Pushcart Press, 1976 - present

CATHEDRAL

AN ILLNESS AND A HEALING

A MEMOIR
BILL HENDERSON

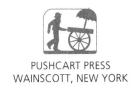

PUSHCART PRESS
WAINSCOTT, NEW YORK

Distributed by WW Norton & Company, Inc
500 Fifth Avenue
New York, NY 10110

Published by Pushcart Press
P.O. Box 380
Wainscott, NY 11975

ISBN 978-1-888889-75-8

*Some portions of Cathedral have appeared elsewhere in
different versions.*

{ FOR GENIE AND LILY }

THIS IS A STORY ABOUT AN AGING MAN
WHO ATTEMPTS TO BUILD A HOLY PLACE
IN HIS BACK YARD.
IT INVOLVES BUGS, LOUSY WEATHER,
CANCER AND SPIRITUAL WAVERINGS.

MY INSPIRATIONS WERE CHARTRES CATHEDRAL,
ST. FRANCIS OF ASSISI,
AND THE FAITH OF FAMILY AND NEIGHBORS.

B. H.

I
{CHARTRES}

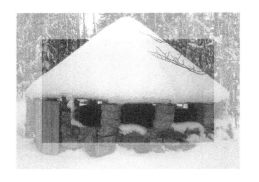

Thin place

BENEATH THE VAULTS OF CHARTRES,
THE ATHEIST WOULD FEEL UNEASY.

Napolean

{THIN PLACE}

*A*fter nine months of writing books and living in poverty in the basement of a Normandy farm house, my wife and I decided we had to leave France, head home and find work. We spent the last of our savings on bus trips to the cathedrals of Beauvais, Rouen, Amiens, Eure, Toulouse and finally Chartres.

Nancy, a recent ex-nun and now angry atheist, was unimpressed by most of the cathedrals. She and her former faith were not on speaking terms. But even she wasn't prepared for that first vision of Chartres.

We had been gazing out the bus window at the flat cornfields of Beauce with little interest when suddenly in the distance we saw something that just shouldn't have been there—an immense edifice, the whole works lifting into the blue sky like an improbable and sudden shout.

As we entered Chartres through the Round Portal we discovered statues of Aristotle, Euclid, Cicero, Boethius, Ptolemy and other ancients (all designated as honorary Christians) among the apostles, and saints who were staring into the distance with open-mouthed amazement or grim determination, some bearing the instruments of their torture. There were also mule-eared devils and their victims being hauled to hell. And, of course, Mary and her son.

Much of the building funds came from tithes and taxes extracted from the common folk, who were honored—or pacified—for their contributions by depiction in the cathedral's windows and statues—weaving and carding wool, harvesting grain, slaughtering livestock and cutting stone.

The soaring sanctuary seemed to ignore its stone pillars. The weightless walls showered the interior with light from small and huge assemblages of stained glass, a glass that has never been duplicated.

A leap to heaven. A grasp for the stars. As a boy I had thrown open my bedroom window in the dark night and stretched out my hands to the infinite. Expecting what? A touch of God's fingertips?

We strive for the Thin Place where the divine and human meet.

Despite our young cynicism, our visit to Chartres in the summer of 1970 took Nancy and me to a very Thin Place.

In following years, Nancy and I divorced. She wrote a book about her convent days and another about her rejection of the Catholic Church. She remarried and divorced again and joined a rebel Catholic organization—the popeless American Catholic Church—which ordained her as a priest.

She died in 1998, a priest.

Days before her death she mailed me a goodbye photo of herself in a sweatshirt. Printed across the front in bold was one word "LOVE."

Many years later, and knowing far less than the master builders of Chartres, I planned my own leap into the sky, with my own honorary Christians in glass and stone. My family, my friends, my neighbors— these would be my honored saints.

I would build my own cathedral on a hill overlooking the sea. I would do this by myself over a long time. I imagined there was no rush. Indeed the idea of rush was anathema to me. Rush was what I had come to this Maine hill to escape.

My cathedral would not imitate Chartres. It would be my own. My "*cathedra*" or bishops seat would be there—as it is in all cathedrals big or small. It is where the bishop sits his butt. My butt.

I would build it as high as I could, using stone found in the woods and blueberry fields, with my own two hands. How high? I had no idea. In fact I'd never laid so much as a brick before, knew nothing about mortar or fitting one rock to another so that the entire pile didn't descend on the worshippers below, but something was going to rise on this 3½ acre lot I owned, and it would be my idea of holy.

We would study there from no single book, no offering would be taken, many hymns would be sung, many prayers uttered (unscripted preferably) but the presiding doctrine would be silence.

This would be a cathedral of shut your mouth and listen.

Listening was easy on that hill. When the wind was still and the birds and crickets and humans and coyotes were sleeping you could hear your ears humming. It was that silent. Visitors from the cities or suburbs found the quiet scary at first. The holy ghost moved about the forests and fields and over the stirring Atlantic and in the distance the eternal mountains sloping to the sea.

One August night in 2002, I sat on my cabin's porch swing with my dog Lulu and watched the full sturgeon moon rise from behind Acadia National Park's mountains, and right beside it was Mars, now a mere 34 million miles from earth, as close as it had been in 60,000 years. The moon broadcast a shimmering path between the sea islands and out to the horizon. Mars was a hot red, and strangely comforting. The solar system had come so close, embracing almost. I looked for the craters of Mars, I waved at Mars. Ridiculously I called "howdy" in the quiet.

And together Mars and the moon continued to rise together, a dance of grace and precision.

Not since 60,000 years—why was I blessed to witness this dance? I wondered.

What had brought me here and what would this hill show me?

"Hello Mars! Hey!" I waved, while my beloved mutt Lulu glanced at me curiously.

"Hey Mars!"

A cathedral on this hill?

Cancer had other plans.

WHAT IS LIFE?
IT IS THE FLASH OF A FIREFLY IN THE
NIGHT.
IT IS THE BREATH OF A BUFFALO IN THE
WINTER TIME.
IT IS THE LITTLE SHADOW THAT RUNS
ACROSS THE GRASS AND LOSES ITSELF IN
THE SUNSET.

Crowfoot

orator of the Blackfoot Nation

{CHRISTY HILL}

*Y*ears ago a real estate agent had mailed me a grainy photo of a lot for sale near a village called Sedgwick on a hill named Christy—Christ with a Y. The local Baptists had been at work with names, I figured. But indeed there had been a Mr. Christy, long gone. His huge farmhouse stood unpainted and aging nearby.

Sedgwick village is at the southern tip of the Blue Hill peninsula that extends into the Atlantic Ocean, bordered on the west by the Penobscot River, which drains much of upstate Maine, and was the conduit for the 19th century logging industry. Long ago Sedgwick was a port town, a hub of the shipbuilding business. Only the old customs house survives from that trade.

You will know you have arrived on the peninsula, because people wave to each other and to strangers as they pass. E. B. White described returning to this area as the "sensation of having received a gift from a true love."

Sedgwick village is about nine miles from White's farm. There's a simple pontoon dock on a small harbor and in the summertime kids fish from the dock and swim in the water, which rarely gets over 60 degrees, except for maybe two weeks at the end of August.

Sedgwick village has a post office, a library that opens a few hours a week, and a dozen houses. There's an ancient, gold-domed, Baptist church (now defunct), and a carpenter's shop in a garage attached to the carpenter's house, several artists' studios, plus a small antique store and the home of a lady who sells "fine hand knit sweaters" which she makes right there.

I drove to Sedgwick from our home on Long Island in February, up an icy dirt road, climbing to I knew not what. I emerged into an expanse of snowy blueberry fields. Three deer raced over the fields, startled by a rare human and his dog. Except for a couple of houses, no one.

And out to the east, endless sea, and to the west endless woods and hills.

I bought the land with the last of my savings and eventually built a cabin and a modest sea-gazing tower there. It was a time of great uncertainty in my life. I needed a tower—but not for reaching out to God's fingertips—a tower "for no reason," I called it.

Since I had been a teenager besotted with Thoreau, I knew that God was more likely to be found in nature than the city. It seemed simple to me and to Thoreau. Cities are about stuff and money. They are busy, noisy, and ephemeral. Words like "lifestyle" apply to cities, although in my 50's boyhood the words had yet to become popular nor did its equally obscene twin "consumer." In nature "grandeur" and "reverence" lived. And so it was on Christy Hill.

Mornings, gazing out to sea as the sun rose shining, too bright to look at, I watched a narrow path between two islands named oddly Gott and Placentia, a corruption of the French word for pleasure. To emerge into the open ocean, one sailed between God and Pleasure. I had no idea of any significance here and I doubt if there is any. (Gott was a guy's name, same as Christy.) For decades an old married couple had lived alone on Gott island through all the seasons. It was rumored he had been in the CIA and fled from the world.

The sea changed constantly from blue to slate gray to not there at all, lost in rolling fog banks and, in summer, smog and haze blown down east from the satanic mills and highways of the east coast and Midwest.

Improbably, a herd of buffalo had been imported to another island out there. The buffalo thrived, but curious tourists often pulled ashore with their kayaks and were threatened and even attacked, and the buffalo went back to where they came from.

From Christy Hill, the sea—eight miles distant—always seemed calm. White caps in windstorms could be spotted only with binoculars. Boats cut no wake I could see from 400 feet in the sky.

Barely I could make out the beach evidence of the rising and falling of the tides. Silently through the days the huge tides moved as they always had, while we the living plotted and planned.

Below my hill a distant church spire thrust itself into the sky. A phallus, a sword, a finger pointing to God—or threatening Him. Who knows what such spires mean. Maybe just a handy place to hang a propaganda bell.

However, according to such spires God is definitely up there. Why up?

My cathedral would do no erecting, pointing, threatening, or ringing. The sky over the mountains, fields and sea already encompassed more glory than any man-made upchuck.

The sun in that sky rose in summer far to the North over Acadia National Park—first light in late June about 3:30 a.m. No sunrise was ever the same. And no day, even the most gray, stayed still for long. The sky was a kaleidoscope of colors rivaling Chartres' windows. Fog gave way to mist and clear blue and pale purple to sunset's bright orange and scarlet. From minute to minute the sky show had no program. Anything could happen and did, with high drama. Except on windy days it was all accomplished in silence.

In the early summer mornings that loud silence was interrupted by mating birds, but by late summer only a lone jay or crow, or the yapping of a coyote convention discussing the latest concerns of neighborhood coyotes, disturbed the morning stillness.

As the temperature rose the bugs did too—black flies in spring, mosquitoes in summer on into the fall. Then I wished only for wind to drive them off so that I could begin work on my cathedral in the deep woods.

Such a breeze often rose from the cold sea as the sun heated the blueberry fields. Unobstructed it surged against Christy Hill and both cooled and deloused the air. Then my dog and I could emerge from the screened porch and walk the deep woods searching for a building sight.

Winds from the west brought more bugs from inland and now and then thunderstorms that piled up over the western mountains, announced by distant and increasingly loud alarms of thunder that drove Lulu under the porch in terror.

Such storms, arriving at my cabin, protected only by a small windbreak of trees were frightening to me too. The tower vibrated as I put my back to it, wondering if it would be driven off its granite ledge.

But the clearing of such storms out to sea was like a quiet prayer. The thunder faded, the late afternoon sun illuminated the departing clouds. I sat stunned watching the raw beauty of it. Often a rainbow arched over all the islands, one end anchored to Acadia's Cadillac Mountain, the other to Swan's Island with Gott and Placentia sheltered under the arch. Out of nothing. This! Hallelujah!

In July all nature held us in its warmth. My visiting wife Annie and daughter Holly slept for ten or more hours at night and napped for another hour in the idyllic afternoons. So deep was our slumber that Annie and I worried that some day we might not be able to wake up.

Only in August did we emerge from our summer hibernation. About the second week, on days when the wind was from the Atlantic, I built the first evening fire in the Franklin stove. By mid-September the first frost threatened and by September's end temperatures in the cool valleys had plummeted and the leaves of the swamp maples were bright red.

Alone now—Annie was back home in Long Island and Holly at school—Lulu and I moved through the woods as huge fog banks rolled in from the sea. I could see them forming far out and watched fascinated as they began to hurry toward Christy Hill at twilight. Suddenly they were upon us. The leaves dripped all night with moisture. In the morning intricate spider webs were a damp gossamer in the grass.

But as summer faded, the skies were usually clear. July's industrial haze was long gone as was mid August's Perseid showers of shooting stars and the distant sails of yachts. The moon and its friend Mars rose from the sea farther to the south. The long twilights of mid-summer sadly shortened.

The crickets began to holler for mates and moved

into the cabin for warmth, as did many spiders and the occasional noisy red squirrel in the attic. Flocks of wild turkeys gleaned the blueberry fields, gobbling and wary of Lulu. Blackbirds swarmed and screeched to each other as if at a New York cocktail party, warming up for their southern migration, hundreds of them in the trees and gone in a flash.

The stars were sharper and brighter in the cold air, their light billions of years old. I looked back in time and imagined God out there. But I knew that God had little to do with stars or moons or up or down. Great distance did not create great spirit—that happened in the human heart. "Love the Lord God with all your heart, soul, mind and strength... and your neighbor as yourself" He said.

No mention of a telescope.

As the sun died that fall and I pondered a cathedral, the garden and field flowers rioted into color—white and red asters, goldenrod, phlox and on the side of the tower, climbing to the very peak, blue and white morning glories.

In the window boxes impatiens and petunias thrived in the chill air and what was left of the garden's turnips, soy beans, pole beans, squash, potatoes, kale, tomatoes, cucumber and lamb's quarter (also known as pig weed—a gift from the wild) fed me.

Through the summer I kept faith with that

garden, and, like Thoreau's faith of the milkweed, the garden—my first ever—had kept faith with me. Since I wanted no electricity or plumbing I collected water from roof run off into pails and when that was gone in dry periods, I filled the pails at nearby Black Pond and drove them, sloshing about, up the hill in my car's open trunk. Each plant had been tended personally by my watering can. Human and dog water was drawn from a hand pump drilled 160 feet down into the hill.

In the woods that would shelter the cathedral, only a few old time beech trees 50 or 60 feet tall—too much bark for the beetles to girdle them—had survived a beech plague. The younger beeches were slowly and horribly dying, a forest of dead stalks. In the still night I now and then heard a crash as one of them gave up. Only the red maples, moose maples, birch and spruce survived. They would inherit these woods when the beeches—joy of Chartres glaziers who treasured them for mixing their window colors—were gone and the beetles moved off to torture other beeches.

It was hard enough for any tree to live long here. Decayed granite was only 2½ feet under the poor soil, no room to feed, let alone anchor. Yet the trees grappled up to the light, wasting not a sun beam, battling each other for what little there was, while all around them lay the rotting hulks.

Through the hardscrabble woods moved turkeys, red squirrels, porcupines, deer, raccoons, fishers, lynx, bears and a reputed mountain lion ("We saw his tail switch behind a bush," said one villager). Everybody treasured a lion, moose or bear sighting. The moose dwelled deep in the woods and were rare hereabouts, but the bears cavorted at bird feeders and in the blueberry fields, scooping up berries and lolling about. The bears were terrified of my gentle Lulu. Hunters were permitted to pursue bears with a pack of up to four hounds. Why kill bear? I never have figured that out. Boredom, I suppose. Maine hunting was a magnet for hunters of all sorts, more than the relic of St. Ann's head was for the Chartres tourists.

Wild animals and citizens were equally wary of hunters. Every fall people clothed themselves in blaze orange hats, vests, sweaters and bustled about daily business like a flock of blazing minstrels. Orange were the leaves and oranger still the locals, afraid they'd be mistaken for fair game as they shopped, walked or drove their cars.

Their fear was not misplaced. Every hunting season somebody was shot by a hunter who just had to kill anything that moved: the most notable victim was a young mother of two kids who was hanging her wash on her backyard line and wearing white gloves. A hunter with a telescopic lens slaughtered her, mistaking the gloves for the tail of a white tailed deer, he said. In two trials he was acquitted. The blame, it seemed to the juries, was on the woman. She was from "away" (Ohio) and didn't know better than to wear white mittens in the fall.

Above the orange forest and the orange humans soared predators with better eyesight than hunters—hawks, kestrels, ospreys and eagles. The eagle is our national bird. Ben Franklin proposed the wild turkey for that symbol. Once at nearby Walker Pond I watched an osprey spear a fish and settle down to lunch. An eagle decided he wanted that fish and he plunged from the sky in ambush. He killed the osprey and filched his fish. I like Ben's bird better. Turkeys take care of each other in their flocks and, to my knowledge, have never murdered, stolen or invaded.

By fall, all the blueberry fields that were bearing fruit that year had been raked by Haitian or Hispanic workers, laughing and calling to each other to pass the hot hours. A few years ago Mainers made a family party out of blueberry raking. No longer. Many fields are owned by large corporations and blueberries are a bottom line business, a keystone of the Maine economy, as is lobster fishing from peninsula harbors.

In early September my daughter and I had ventured into the fields to glean what the bears and rakers had missed. We cooked blueberry pancakes one Sunday morning, our last breakfast together before

Holly returned to school.

The blueberry fields gradually turned to maroon. Large trucks packed with hay bales were unloaded and hay was spread over the fields for burning, a pest control ritual dating back centuries.

Past the western fields mist rose on cold mornings from Black and Grey Ponds and further off the mighty Penobscot River, once jammed with logs for the mills along its shore, moved down from the northern forest. Now logs were trucked and trained to the one local mill at Bucksport where coated paper was prepared for junk glossies in New York like *People*.

To the east, past Brooklin Village ("boat building capital of the world") to the ocean shores, the air roared with chain saws as orange clad figures stocked in the 6 or 7 cords necessary to survive the long winter ahead.

On Sedgwick's Benjamin River harbor, the pleasure yachts were hauled out to be wrapped in plastic for the winter and along Eggemoggin Reach between Sedgwick and Deer Isle, the old-time gaff-rigged multi-masted touring sailboats (more barges than yachts) had given up the tourist trade until next summer.

Before Holly left for school we had scouted the woods for a cathedral site. Nothing seemed special—flat and featureless. But in one spruce copse,

Holly came upon a small rock outcropping. "It just felt right" Holly said later. She began to peel back the rock's moss cover. I joined in and we soon realized that this was no piddling stone but a substantial boulder.

We set to work with a pick ax, shovel, hammer and saw and soon uncovered a relatively flat oval ledge, cracked in the middle like a broken heart. The break between the two halves of the heart formed a natural pew on one side and an altar on the other.

This spot, alone in the woods, seemed miraculous to Holly and me—the perfect cathedral foundation. Until now this ledge had never seen the light, perhaps for thousands of years.

Words cannot touch what that foundation meant to us. Something holy had been buried and resurrected.

Long after Holly had left and Annie had returned to Long Island, I sat in my stone pew, my arm around Lulu. We were alone now and would be here until the first freeze, and the second and third freeze. Until we could take the cold no longer in the summer cabin and would flee south.

II
{How To}

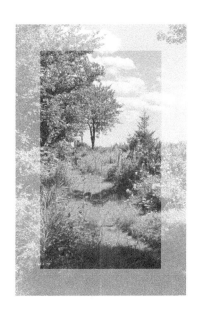

WHAT WE DO NOT COMPREHEND, AND
NEVER SHALL, IS THE APPETITE BEHIND
ALL THIS; THE GREED FOR NOVELTY:
THE FUN OF LIFE.

Henry Adams
Mt. St. Michel & Chartres

{THE TREBUCHET}

*V*ictor Hugo remarked that Romanesque churches sat squat and somber "as if crushed" —massive walls, heavy roofs, stifling dark. The entire weight of medieval theological doctrine weighed on the helpless worshippers.

The sudden inspiration of the Gothic changed all that. In Chartres a new world vision was imagined for the first time since the fall of Rome. Chartres was not intended as art, but as a representation of the universe, a moral reality and evocation of the heavenly city.

Chartres' beauty is not achieved because its designers considered themselves to be designers of perfection. In fact, part of the impact of Chartres is its very imperfection. The unequal spires, the slanting floor, the slightly off center Royal Portal and countless other mistakes that only prove that human beings—sinners, if you will—fashioned this building, often without complete plans and by the seat of their pants.

(King Solomon, it might be noted, knew exactly what he wanted for his temple—"Sixty cubits long, twenty cubits wide and thirty cubits high...when the house was built, it was with stone prepared at the quarry, so that neither hammer nor axe nor any tool of iron was heard in the temple." 1 Kings).

After the rocks were lugged to Chartres, the problem was how to pile them up. Here the bloody craftiness of war joined the holy craft of the master builders.

A deadly device called the *trebuchet*, a kind of catapult, used counterweights to toss missiles of up to 300 pounds for hundreds of feet and splatter infidels. God and war intoxications were linked when the modified *trebuchet* was employed to raise Chartres' stone walls.

The master builders had other unique problems: for instance how to fashion the new cathedral with the remains of a 1194 fire. The surviving structures were obviously blessed by the Virgin Mary who saved them. They couldn't be torn down. Therefore the nave had to be fitted to them somehow. The result is a nave that doesn't merge with the west end, it smashes into it.

New foundations were required on the site of the burned hulk. A miscalculation here would topple all that followed. After the foundations the outer walls were erected and supported with the beams and the marvelous invention of flying buttresses.

Meanwhile worshippers and tourists sought the holy in the midst of hundreds of swarming workers, piles of scrap and stone, gigantic machines and constant racket and clatter.

Chartres was always open for business.

Essential to all this was mortar—a combination of chalk that had been crushed and baked to form quicklime and then slaked with water and mixed with sand to form a putty. Mortar took a while to set, even years. But unlike the mortar I later used on Christy Hill, it would reset itself if disturbed by shifts in wall mass.

Because of the unusually warm climate in Europe, the mortar could be applied in all but the coldest months, perhaps another blessing from Mary.

Stone, then mortar, stone then mortar—Chartres climbed towards God's throne. To get to the upper reaches, the master builders ordered combinations of levers, block and tackles, winches and windlasses, and of course the *trebuchet*.

Since the largest stones could not be lifted all the way up by any other device, they were hoisted by another curious combination—cranes powered by an eight foot in diameter hamster wheel turned by the foot energy of men inside the wheel. One man could raise ten times his own body weight. These odd contraptions might measure more than twenty feet in diameter and enclose several workers. The human hamsters had to precisely orchestrate their deliberate march. To slip meant disaster—the wheel would reverse, drop its load and twirl violently backward, injuring or killing those inside.

Thus did high walls and spires emerge over the fields of Beauce.

On October 24, 1260 it was done. Chartres was completed.

TAKE THAT ROCK OVER THERE, IT DOESN'T SEEM TO BE DOING MUCH OF ANYTHING, AT LEAST TO OUR GROSS PERCEPTION. BUT AT THE MICROLEVEL IT CONSISTS OF AN UNIMAGINABLE NUMBER OF ATOMS CONNECTED BY SPRINGY CHEMICAL BONDS, ALL JIGGLING AROUND AT A RATE THAT EVEN OUR FASTEST SUPERCOMPUTER MIGHT ENVY… YOU MIGHT THINK OF THE ROCK AS A PURELY CONTEMPLATIVE BEING. AND YOU MIGHT DRAW THE MORAL THAT THE UNIVERSE IS, AND ALWAYS HAS BEEN, SATURATED WITH MIND.

Jim Holt

{ ROCKS }

To build a stone cathedral you need a nearby supply of rocks. Since Downeast Maine is mostly all rocks—with some gravel sprinkled here and there—that should have been no problem.

On my few acres, the rocks were everywhere, most obviously in the stone wall at the edge of the property, huge rocks, dug from the blueberry fields and roughly stacked to mark property lines centuries ago—a job for teams of horses and many men. But for the lone cathedral builder, those rocks were impossible to budge, let alone haul or roll to the site that Holly and I had clawed from the forest floor.

The roadsides, fields and woods were strewn with all manner of rocks. The beach at Sedgwick harbor and on Eggemoggin Reach had collected eons of pebbles and small transportable stones. But all of these rocks were of little use because they were lopsided—flat on one side, and crazy on the other, triangulated, perfectly round, pointy, bumpy—in short, any possible shape except flat.

Since I was too broke to hire a mason to help me, I determined to let common sense be my rule: use only rocks found in nature; let gravity do the work. Common sense said if rocks were relatively flat on two sides and well balanced and placed, then they would stay up. Gravity was my friend.

Mortar I wasn't too sure about, although it was cheap and easy to come by. The Deer Isle lumber yard sold mortar makings in 40 and 80 pound bags, ready to mix with water. Presto, glue for rocks. But my friend A.J. Billings, owner of the yard, could promise only 50 years of durability—"After that, mortar cracks and decays." said A.J. In answer to my curious question about an eternal monument A.J. allowed "You're much better off making sure the walls are plumb and well stacked. Gravity will hold those rocks on top of each other for a heck of a long time."

A.J. taught me all I know about building, and he was ready with his Maine humor, too, comparing me to Tom Sawyer in the woods and joking about my edifices blowing down with me on them.

My only problem was that flat-on-two-opposite sides rocks are as rare in nature as a cuddly porcupine. Nowhere in woods or fields did I find more than one or two candidates that were suitably two sided and that I could lift (60 pounds max) to my wheel barrow or beat-up car and transport to the foundation ledge.

What saved my cathedral was the several abandoned quarries near the hill, some down long, rutted woods roads, others, such as the one at the end of Radar Road, relatively easy to get to with the car and well-stocked with leftover shards of rocks,

blasted and rejected for buildings, roads or bridges.
Down the Radar Road Lulu and I walked most
days, rock hunting. We passed the decrepit Radar
Station, built about the year I was born, now just
a 20 x 40 foot pile of cement blocks painted yellow
long ago and used as a storage barn. Next to the
Radar Station were the buried pilings and anchor
bolts for the long deceased radar tower, the bolts
reaching only inches into the sky. During World War
II the station was constantly manned to search the
sea for Nazi submarines. Now it was a gloomy hulk,
a tombstone planted on top of Christy Hill and left
to crumble.

A short way down Radar Road to the quarry
was a section compulsively posted with instructions,
often two or three to a tree every 100 feet or so:
"No Hunting" "No Trapping" "No Trespassing"
"Sky Ledge Sanctuary" "Private Road" "Violators
will be Prosecuted" "Report Violations to Wildlife
Land Trust, The Humane Society of the United
States."

Those signs were the work of a nearby recluse,
who lived with his mother down a dirt road in an
old house. I'd never seen anybody near that house.
It was lifeless. But his signs sang out for him. The
neighbors said he loved black bears, that he had
names for all the bears for miles around; that when
one was killed, injured, or shot, he wept. "They shot
Curly," "Baby's been hit by a car!" he'd announce

to whomever he met.

Years later he tried to commit suicide with a long swim in February waters. A cop rescued him at the last minute. "Zygote" they called him.

A part of me felt deeply for Zygote. As a boy I had plastered trees in the woods behind our Philadelphia suburban house with signs—"No Hunting Allowed," "Predator Hunting OK"—and signed them "The Henderson Game Commission." What I meant was, you can kill the mean foxes and crows, but spare the bunnies and deer. Moral messages for a minuscule forest. Never mind that the last deer had disappeared from that suburb years ago and there was little left to hunt. My posters flapped in an empty woods. Soon the woods disappeared. A housing development wiped out even the remaining bunnies.

About a mile past the Radar Station and the Hunting Forbidden Zone, was Dave Webb's quarry—piles of pea stone, gravel and various rip rap, plus now and then a stone with two opposite sides flat. I piled these treasures by the road to return later with the car, while Lulu swam with abandon in the quarry's many ponds.

This quarry was about much more than just rocks. Various paths led to brush dumps, the sites of summertime parties—piles of empty beer cans and burned logs, and a wrecked car pulverized with bullet holes and surrounded by broken glass, plastic kids' toys, a play pen, baby bottles and broken furniture as if some crazed spouse had dumped his car and family and fled. On a rock entrance to this path a spray painted message mysteriously pronounced "It's 4:16 and only a minute to go," and nearby "Burn the Man."

High piles of bulldozed blueberry fields surrounded this wreckage. But I didn't mourn the destroyed fields. Here I might find more gravity friendly rocks, something of value. One day in eternity the blueberries would reclaim all this.

I THINK I COULD TURN AND LIVE WITH
ANIMALS, THEY'RE SO PLACID AND SELF-
CONTAIN'D. I STAND AND LOOK AT THEM
LONG AND LONG. THEY DO NOT SWEAT
AND WHINE ABOUT THEIR CONDITION,
THEY DO NOT LIE AWAKE IN THE DARK AND
WEEP FOR THEIR SINS, THEY DO NOT MAKE
ME SICK DISCUSSING THEIR DUTY TO GOD.

Walt Whitman

{ LULU }

When my dog Lulu was diagnosed with cancer, about the same time I was, some people, including my oncologist, found my depression over her dying hard to understand. It's just a dog, I heard in their muted expression of sympathy.

But Lulu was more than just a dog. I talked to her like a comrade, since the first day I adopted her from the local animal shelter, where she had languished for over a year.

Lulu was ninety pounds of shaggy mutt. In fact, her shelter name had been Chewy, after the hairy *Star Wars* character. She looked as if a committee had tacked her together, with a German shepherd face, floppy dreadlocked Airedale ears, and a Golden Retriever body. Her muzzle said ferocious, her eyes indicated kind, and her tail wagged like a puppy's for friend and stranger alike.

Our delight during our ten years together was the Long Island bay beaches in winter and the Maine woods in summer and fall. Lulu, with her long coat, hated heat; she adored snow and ice. In January she'd plunge into the surf with a gigantic happy splash—and paddle past ice flows to retrieve sticks I had tossed.

In the summer, after a day curled under the

cabin's porch to avoid the heat, she emerged at sunset for our ritual evening tennis ball game on our ridge road overlooking the sea. Until old age and cancer slowed her down, she chased balls into the twilight and then we both crashed in the grass and felt the darkness fall around us.

Lulu would jump on the sofa when I seemed depressed, rest her head on my shoulder, and stay that way, or lick my hand until I told her enough already. When other dogs rushed up to us snarling and threatening, she calmed them with her steady gaze and firm but pacific stand.

Lulu and I were kids together. We pretended we were not aged ten and sixty plus. We would romp forever. Or I pretended and Lulu just couldn't be bothered with age.

One last disease-free golden October, Lulu and I sat at the cathedral site and watched the sun rise through the trees. No walls had been raised, the ledge was still our cathedral and our sanctuary—open for business.

Each morning was our sacred moment before the day broke in profane shatter around us, a distant truck or school bus humming dimly or a jet darting toward Bar Harbor airport.

As a breeze stirred the spruces I recited my one prayer "God of love and wonder, grant me the grace to remember you today and let me live my life as a prayer to you."

And listening to the silence, I'd wait for wordless grace to descend. Always the rising sun was enough. Lulu on the rock beside me, her head on her paws, had no need for grace.

I breathed deep gulps to still my monkey mind. What I sought was beyond words—even the words "love" and "wonder." So I forgot the words and sat wordless with wordless Lulu.

One morning Lulu stood in the new sunlight in front of me on the altar rock. She stared me full in the face, her eyes large and concentrating on me as I sat on the ledge's pew. "Are you God?" I asked her. Like God, she did not immediately reply, just curled up next to me seeming to feel what I tried to feel, holy stillness. For her it was easier, she had no words spinning through her brain.

Wasn't it odd, I thought afterward, I sought the same wordless faith that I had criticized my Pop for. When I belligerently asked Pop to detail the reasons for his belief that Jesus is Lord, for his constant prayer through the day, for his diligent tithing and church attendance, he dismissed me—"If you don't know by now, I can't tell you."

Pop spent his entire adult life, almost four decades, traveling for the General Electric Company as an engineer in charge of repairing low-voltage industrial switch gear.

On his trips, Pop was addicted to the frightful radio bombast of evangelists Carl McIntire and Oral

Roberts, who preached fire and damnation for communists and other nonbelievers and heavenly bliss for the likes of Pop and his family. In order to be sure I was safe from God's furnace, I missed not one Sunday for over a decade, starting in nursery school. I was awarded a gold bar for every one of those years. The string of bars was stuck right there on the lapel of my sports jacket: a perfect record, and one of the longest periods of Sunday school attendance in the recent history of the national Presbyterian Church.

Pop was certain about eternal burnings for the unsaved dead, but he was incredibly tender to all living beings. He never struck me in anger, and the only time he accidentally smacked me he fell into spasms of apology. He was so gentle that he refused to prune live limbs on trees in our backyard. During our annual one-day summer fishing trip on the Ocean City, New Jersey bay, he wouldn't bait his hooks with live minnows. Instead, he brought along frozen clam strip bait and was quite happy to catch nothing at all. I gladly skewered the squirming minnows and hoped for a prize flounder.

I think Pop would have liked to become an evangelist, but he was too agonizingly shy. After he died, on one of the few scraps of paper he left behind from his college days, I found this resolve to himself: "Have fellowship with whomever you meet and witness the love of God which passes understanding…" But when guests appeared at the door to our house, Pop fled to his basement workshop and let Mom handle the chin music.

"If you don't know by now, I can't tell you"—words wouldn't help.

I used to think this was a cop out, a dodge to get rid of his pestering adolescent son, who had become enamored with Kant, Neitzche, Schopenhauer, et al. in Will Durant's popular history *The Story of Philosophy*, my new Bible.

Here I was on this ledge with Lulu, seeking not a philosophic word gaggle, but the same quiet faith Pop had known.

In our last night together that summer Holly, Annie and I held hands around the porch dinner table. No words to our prayer. Our touch was that prayer. Holly was the priest—only when she squeezed Annie's and my hands would the silence end and the circle be broken.

Now, with my arm around Lulu I recalled that parting silence.

"Are you God?" I repeated.

Lulu laughed and jumped off the altar. It was time to hunt rocks.

YOU HAVE NOTICED THAT EVERY THING
THE INDIAN DOES IS IN A CIRCLE, AND
THAT IS BECAUSE THE POWER OF THE
WORLD MOVES IN CIRCLES AND EVERY
THING TRIES TO BE ROUND...

Black Elk

{ ROUND }

*D*reaming of my cathedral had urged me through that first doubting winter.

I remembered a notice posted at the Brooklin Store: "Field rocks at $40 a ton, Delivered." Maybe in the spring it would be possible to find at least a few flat rocks in such a ton. This rock hunt with my rock hound was never going to discover enough suitable stone for a worthy edifice.

It was a winter of dismissals—a book proposal about my favorite hymns had been rejected by my previous publisher; various colleges ignored my employment applications; Guggenheim and National Endowment grants were declined; an attempt to start an endowment for the Pushcart Prize, a celebration of small press authors, was going nowhere and sales of the Pushcart Prize, a book I had published every year since 1976, featuring thousands of short stories, essays and poems, were slipping in the wake of the 9/11 World Trade Center attack and the recession that followed. In fact, The Pushcart Prize was finished unless major benefactors appeared or I found a job—an impossibility for a guy at retirement age.

I was bereft of plans, a failure on every front, despair close at hand. In my 8 x 8' shack of an office in our Long Island back yard I had long ago posted a monk's advice: "Despair is an aspect of pride." But I usually forgot the note was there, as I slogged on into a spring and summer of uncertainty.

Of rocks I was sure. "On this rock I will build my church." Peter was that fallible rock, tradition said, a most unworthy rock. Me too, and I was surrounded by unworthy stones. They would have to do.

But what shape the cathedral? A modified cross like Chartres? No. Round. It had to be round. All the churches of my youth had been rectangles—the simple summer chapel in Ocean City, New Jersey; the pretentious boxed Bryn Mawr Presbyterian church in suburban Philadelphia where, of a Sunday, Rolls Royces and their chauffeurs waited for their worshipping bosses.

In such chapels and churches I had learned a boxed doctrine. Heaven is for the saved (us)— everybody else burns forever. A tidy package as long as you didn't try to exit the box.

A round structure implied an eternal circle of questions. There would be no neat corners for cute theology in a round cathedral. Besides, the box is unnatural. In nature there were few boxes—the moon, the sun, the earth, tree trunks, all round. A box was an anathema in all I saw around me.

I imagined the cathedral with high windows— stained glass of my own making perhaps. Definitely no Gothic buttresses, gables, colonettes, gargoyles, pinnacles, crockets, trefoils, quatrefoils or cinque-foils. But a rock floor for sure, (already installed) and maybe a candle to symbolize the fire that is life—"every common bush afire with God" as Elizabeth Barrett Browning observed.

And a cross? Probably not. Too specific of past spoiled doctrine, like jewelry around a starlet's neck or the cross handle of Constantine's sword—"By this sign I will triumph!" A torture device. The cross—the most abused symbol in history. Yet for me it still meant the unfathomable love of one rebel for all of us living, dead, and still to come. I'd have to ponder a cross.

But round was for sure. It was revealed, slowly, under the hardscrabble that Holly and I had hacked away—the round, broken heart. I am still amazed by what Holly and I found on those late summer days when sea winds swept the mosquitoes from the woods and let us tear at the earth in peace.

Holly approved of my round concept. Her's was a round theology. At college in Northampton, Massachusetts she attended both a Quaker meeting and a Unitarian Church. "That makes me a Quackertarian," she smiled.

No boxes there.

WHEN A FRIEND CALLS TO ME
FROM THE ROAD AND SLOWS
HIS HORSE TO A MEANING
WALK, I DON'T STAND STILL
AND LOOK AROUND ON ALL
THE HILLS I HAVEN'T HOED,
AND SHOUT FROM WHERE I AM,
"WHAT IS IT?"... I THRUST MY
HOE IN THE MELLOW GROUND,
BLADE-END UP AND FIVE FEET
TALL, AND PLOD:
I GO UP TO THE STONE WALL
FOR A FRIENDLY VISIT.

Robert Frost

{ NEIGHBORS }

*I*t's tough to keep a secret in Sedgwick village. Obviously through the summers something was going on back in the woods. All those rocks piled up by the road; the man from away, and sometimes his daughter, emerging from the woods sweating and hauling more rocks.

I welcomed neighbors' visits and tried to explain the mystery of what I intended. I had yet to tell the town's building code inspector. Town rules asked only to be informed if a structure was to be in excess of 75 square feet. Lousy at math and round measurements I had no idea where I was going with square footage, so I laid low.

My visitors understood "cathedral," but me they had a hard time figuring out—particularly on the day I had dropped a huge dying birch tree right next to the sacred ledge. I used no power tools in any of my projects. I had gone after this giant with a tree handsaw, barely wide enough to get through its trunk. I'd tied off the birch to a nearby moose maple and, in case it plummeted down on me, I planned my escape path to the other side of the maple.

With trepidation I began to cut a notch away from the ledge, in the direction I wanted the tree to topple. Birches are heavy, filled with sap, even if half dead. And they have few branches to catch on other trees, so they free-fall fast and hard. You don't want to be near a big falling birch alone in the woods. As I approached my notch from the other side, I got ready to run. At the first crack of splitting wood I dashed for the exit—then louder pops and soon the giant was down explosively.

And I was safe.

My immediate thought, besides relief, was what a genius I was. I'd dropped it exactly away from the ledge as I had intended, with a handsaw. Me and my little saw had felled a Goliath.

Elated I headed back through the woods for a drink of cool water from the pump. And suddenly I found myself on the forest floor, my right knee smashed and bleeding. Dumbfounded, I couldn't figure out what had hit me. I thought my building days were ended. But I could still painfully limp. I bandaged up the knee and later hobbled back to the path to find what I had tripped over.

Nothing.

No stump. No rock. No hole. The path was smooth. There was utterly no reason for my fall—except, I concluded, hubris. What I had tripped over—that invisible stump or stone or hole—I called God's Stumbling Block, a reminder that just because I could pinpoint drop that tree with a hand-saw, I was not such a hot shot after all.

Through the woods that day came two

neighbors—Jean Hendrick and Jill Knowles—out for a bike ride. We inspected my cathedral site and during iced tea on the porch, I explained my hubris theory of the smashed knee. "That's interesting" they allowed, obviously wary of my mind's working. Perhaps a concussion? Chopping down a tree and he gets a celestial whacking? With tight smiles, they thanked me for the tea, wished a quick recovery, and pedaled down the hill.

Years later I remain convinced that something had felled me for my hubris. But I never found out what, other than the outraged hand of God.

IN THIS SAME YEAR MEN FIRST BEGAN TO HARNESS THEMSELVES AND DRAG TO CHARTRES CARTS LOADED WITH STONES AND TIMBERS, CORN AND OTHER THINGS TO HELP TOWARD THE BUILDING OF THE CHURCH, WHOSE TOWERS WERE THEN BEING CONSTRUCTED. YOU COULD HAVE SEEN MEN AND WOMEN MOVING ON THEIR KNEES THROUGH THICK MUD, AND BEING BEATEN WITH SCOURGES, MANY MIRACLES HAPPENING ALL OVER THE PLACE, CHANTS AND HYMNS OF JOY BEING OFFERED TO GOD.

Robert of Torigni
Abbot of St. Michel

*M*ost of that second summer Lulu and I collected rocks, a respectable heap of them.

To layout my circular cathedral I positioned a stick between the altar and the pew stones in the crevice of the broken heart. I ran a 12 foot string around a circle, marking the circumference with pebbles. That would be the outside wall. How wide and how high I'd figure out later.

Then I began.

Living the Good Life, by Helen and Scott Nearing, a stone besotted testament, was my Bible. A whole generation of back-to-the-landers had migrated to this peninsula in the 60's and 70's, in thrall to the Nearings, who built in stone—even their garden fences were rock—and lived off the land through the bitter Maine winters.

From the Nearings I learned I needed to clean my stones, a thorough scrubbing with a wire brush on each surface to be mortared. Each stone should also be mudded (slapped upon with mortar). For this rubber gloves were a necessity since mortar burned the skin.

I hauled my water to the site in buckets filled from cisterns of roof run off. Dry mortar was stored in a plastic tub by the road and mixed in small, one rock batches. As my friend A.J. of the Deer Isle lumberyard counseled, it was important to maintain a thick, almost dry—definitely not wet—consistency. Mix it wrong and it wouldn't set correctly. Mix it at air temperatures below 50° and it would never set up.

Some nights the night air hit 45°—too cold. The next day it backed into the 50's but those nights may be the reason why, when I tested a few of my first circle rocks a year later, they all dislodged from the ledge as if never mortared at all. But that second September, I didn't know this would happen.

I had a few days to close the first circle before the next temperature drop. Mercifully, the mosquitoes were long gone by now. We could work at will.

Lulu and I hustled off to new abandoned quarries and picked up flat-on-two-sides rocks with urgency. We found dirt-bike paths that led to slag piles, and ponds for Lulu to swim in, laughing, tongue-out happy.

Odd parties had gone on back down those paths. The celebrants had left behind burned logs in a square around a doll, an outlined penis, and "Hell is Here" spray painted on boulders.

Usually nobody was in the quarries, but one day a guy on Dave Webb's land was loading gravel into a dump truck. I waved at him. He didn't wave back. This was not typical. In Sedgwick everybody waved, at passing cars, or joggers or pedestrians or rare birds in noontime quarries. Strangers and neighbors and friends all received at least a few raised fingers on the steering wheel.

No wave from the big guy of the quarry. I shouldn't be there, I imagined he was thinking. The dog was probably just a cover for nefarious deeds. I was trespassing.

After he left, Lulu and I returned in the wheezing Volvo to pick up the six rocks we had prospected and rushed them back to the ledge as the September sun neared the tree line in the southwest.

The altar dipped to the heart's center a bit. Here two-sided flat rocks were not required—only the top needed to be flat and the bottom sloping to make up for the altar's dip. I had several stones that worked out fine there. I mortared them in as yellow and red leaves began to cover the altar like a fiery blanket against the coming winter.

I placed the last stone in the first circle and headed to the Buck's Harbor pub to celebrate. At the bar sat my friend Eliot Coleman, founder and proprietor, with his wife Barbara Damrosch, of Four Seasons Farm near the Nearings holdings.

Eliot told me the story of an old man who had just delivered a truck load of hay to his farm. The old man had a helper, a son of slow mind, who worked in slow motion. He was often abused by other kids at school, Eliot said. His dad labored beside him. His boy was his whole world.

All afternoon the two slowly unloaded the small truck.

"Kindness is all," said Eliot.

TO SAY THAT GOD CAN ONLY TRULY BE
REVEALED IN SCRIPTURE, AS MANY HAVE
INSISTED THROUGH THE AGES, IS A LITTLE
LIKE SAYING THAT, EVEN IF YOU LIVE
RIGHT ACROSS THE STREET FROM THE
BALL PARK WITH A LIFETIME FREE PASS,
THE BEST WAY TO FOLLOW THE YANKEES IS
TO READ ABOUT THEM IN THE PAPERS...

Rev. Rob McCall

My encounter with the sullen stranger in Dave Webb's quarry had raised a question —whose rocks were these anyway? And who owned the abandoned quarries? Should I be paying for my miniscule hauls?

Dave transported gravel, sand and stone by the multi-ton. I'm sure he couldn't care if I scavenged his land. But to be sure—in rising guilt—I went to see him in his village home.

I'd known Dave since my tower building days. When I couldn't dig my foundation tubes deep enough into the hard earth—4 feet minimum was the rule to avoid frost heaves—I hired Dave and his backhoe to help. Through the fragile and dying beech woods he'd crashed with his monster machine and clawed out trenches.

But the earth defeated us both. He couldn't dig deeper than 2½ feet also. The decayed granite crust was just below the surface. Later, as with the cathedral, I discovered a miraculous flat ledge and built my tower there—the Big Bang Boulder I lovingly christened it.

Now Dave and I had other rock business. I approached his house late in the afternoon with apprehension. Maybe the sullen guy had reported me for the trespassing and stealing. Maybe Dave would sneer at me with righteous scorn. Or call the sheriff. Dave held the future of my cathedral in his hands. He was the flat rock king.

Dave, a big, friendly guy, opened his door. "Hi, Bill!"

I blurted out my business. Can I buy a few rocks from you? I find them here and there in your quarry."

"How many rocks do you need, Bill?"

"Maybe a few dozen."

"Sure! Can I help you out? Deliver them?"

"No thanks. I've got the car."

"OK"

"I was wondering how much you want for the rocks?"

"Oh, I dunno, you name it, Bill."

"Buck a rock?" I tried, uncertain if that was far too cheap and he'd send me packing.

"Sure, that's fine."

We said goodbye; he went into his 5:30 p.m. Maine dinner, and I walked home with Lulu, elated.

Suddenly I found myself talking out loud, praying mightily. I'd been given the OK by the Power, Lord of the Flat Rocks—the Keeper of the Keys! "Thank you!" I shouted to the woods, as Lulu and I climbed Christy Hill. Lulu, stopping to pee, shot me her quizzical eye.

I counted my pile—84 rocks, not all of them from Dave's quarry, many of them from the wild.

But I had no exact count. I wrote him a check for $84, noted on the check "as agreed, buck a rock" and carried it down to him.

VAST, TITANIC, INHUMAN NATURE HAS GOT [MAN] AT DISADVANTAGE, CAUGHT HIM ALONE, AND PILFERS HIM OF SOME OF HIS DIVINE FACULTY... SHE SEEMS TO SAY STERNLY, WHY CAME YE HERE BEFORE YOUR TIME? THIS GROUND IS NOT PREPARED FOR YOU... SHOULDST THOU FREEZE OR STARVE OR SHUDDER THY LIFE AWAY, HERE IS NO SHRINE, NOR ALTAR, NOR ANY ACCESS TO MY EAR.

Henry Thoreau
on climbing Maine's Mt. Katahdin (1846)

I was desperate to get at least a start on the second tier of rocks before the first frost. That tier was a much tougher job than laying stone on the mostly flat ledge. No rock was completely flat and each bottom rock and the one to be filled on top of it had its own peculiarities. Fitting them together was like solving a puzzle. I hated puzzles.

I had to wait through the day until the air and rock temperatures rose. The rocks baked in the sun, reaching what I guessed was 50°. Starting at about 2 pm on a typical afternoon I could manage to set only a few in bed with each other, joined by gravity and a slap of mortar mixed with hot water from the cabin stove.

I covered the rocks with a piece of tarpaulin to keep the heat in and the rain out. Copious rain within 24 hours of setting mortar was fatal. It washed the mortar away in a stream. However it was crucial to keep the mortar damp to help it set up—a daily sprinkle through the week.

But that late September—usually a dry period— as I raced to add the second row, it didn't merely sprinkle non-stop; it deluged. Temperatures dropped so suddenly that I had to break off my cathedral labors to cut wood for the woodstove.

"Chop wood, carry water" advised a Zen master to restless monks seeking peace. It didn't work for me. There are few more boring jobs than cutting logs to length with a handsaw and splitting them. I preferred to stay in bed under a mound of blankets. The Holy Spirit was forgotten. I had a cold mind with rocks in it.

Lulu and I found a few more treasures in Dave's quarry but the road was mostly washed out and threatened to pitch the car into a ravine. We sat in the cabin hoping for the weather to clear, dejectedly watching the annual assembly of cluster flies at the window and lady bugs—little gems—scuttling across the sill.

From the dirt road a loud whistle in the early morning damp—it set Lulu to barking and me to rushing to the porch to holler "Good morning, Paul!"

"Morning, Bill" Paul Sullivan yelled back from his yellow-ponchoed hike with his hound Jemima. And indeed it became a good morning.

Paul, a diabetic, was hiking to save his life. If he didn't keep moving the diabetes would kill him.

He was also one of the happiest people on the peninsula—always a glad word for everybody at the general store, post office, church, or hiking with Jemima. When Paul entered a room the place lit up.

Paul, a celebrated composer, played keyboard with the Paul Winter band and for this would win a Grammy. Winter and Sullivan and company performed at the Dodge Poetry Festival, the Winter Solstice Celebration in New York and various gigs on the peninsula and around the world from Siberia to Japan.

Paul's loving piano compositions about Down East Maine, issued on CDs produced at his River Music studios, play in the background as I write this little book. We were brothers in spirit, laughter and idea.

But music aside, what distinguished Paul was his leadership of the local Boy Scout troop, where his son Henry would earn the rank of Eagle Scout amidst a raft of merit badges and congratulatory letters from various politicians. Paul's own scout leadership uniform was festooned with gala ribbons and signals of rank—a mini-general in the pacifist cause.

Unlike Henry, I never progressed beyond First Class Scout, but pegging up a tent, ditching a latrine and sparking a fire with two twigs, led me to a hunger for the wild, and from there to Thoreau and thus to the Maine woods, where on a dripping, shivering morning my favorite Scout master whistled Good Morning to me and Lulu and lifted us from a grand funk.

YOUR RELIGION WAS WRITTEN ON
TABLES OF STONE BY THE IRON
FINGER OF YOUR GOD SO THAT
YOU COULD NOT FORGET.
OUR RELIGION IS THE TRADITIONS
OF OUR ANCESTORS...
WHEN THE LAST RED MAN SHALL
HAVE PERISHED, THESE SHORES
WILL SWARM WITH THE INVISIBLE
DEAD OF MY TRIBE, AND WHEN
YOUR CHILDREN'S CHILDREN
THINK THEMSELVES ALONE IN THE
FIELD, THE STORE, OR IN THE
SILENCE OF THE PATHLESS WOODS,
THEY WILL NOT BE ALONE.

Chief Seattle
1855

*D*epression was never far off in those final days of the second summer of construction. The trees were stripped of their leaves, the ferns dried brown, the crickets quieted. Only the crows found something to laugh about.

I waited for one or two warm days to place one or two new rocks at the cathedral, but I wondered, what was the point of all this?

Why did I need a structure to worship in? Lulu and I were doing fine with our morning meditations on the simple ledge. Other people recognized its holiness. My neighbor Fran Eastman, a tapestry artist and seamstress, had visited the day before. She called the ledge "a very special place," without prompting from me.

How more special would it be with walls and a roof? Indeed I found it hard to pray in many edifices—for instance massive St. John's Cathedral in New York—more mass than soul. Many churches smacked of human ambition. They summoned God into vaulted pretensions. Was I trying to hallow these woods with my own conceit?

Worse, I questioned my own spirit. "God's boy" I sneered at myself. I sat at this broken hearted ledge each day before my mind dissolved back into busyness—had to do that, had to be there. Holy Spirit not even a notion. God's boy was mostly a fraud, I figured, and he shouldn't be raising structures that pretended to be holy.

The cold rain from the sea continued. Lulu and I were soaked and chilled. I was coming down with a cough, a sniffle—the usual mess of winter.

I called Holly at college to give her the depressing update on our project.

"You've got to keep on, Dad. You really want to do this. Forget about your excuses. Just do it," she said.

On the altar I mortared the final stone of the summer—the Holly Stone. Around this rock I'd build my cathedral next spring.

GEESE APPEAR HIGH OVER US,
PASS, AND THE SKY CLOSES. ABANDON,
AS IN LOVE OR SLEEP, HOLDS
THEM TO THEIR WAY, CLEAR,
IN THE ANCIENT FAITH: WHAT WE NEED
IS HERE. AND WE PRAY, NOT
FOR NEW EARTH OR HEAVEN, BUT TO BE
QUIET IN HEART, AND IN EYE
CLEAR. WHAT WE NEED IS HERE.

Wendell Berry
from "The Wild Geese"

{MR. POTATO HEAD}

From Holly I had learned what little I knew. When Holly was very young I tried to tell her about the Jesus I heard about when I was her age, but then she reversed the message and began to teach me.

I tried to explain Christmas to her. "It's a birthday party for a man named Jesus who lived long ago and said we should all love each other," I said, choking.

Concerned by my sadness, and hoping to cheer up me and Jesus, Holly said, "We could get him a Mr. Potato Head for his birthday."

While Holly learned about words like "Jesus" and "Christmas" from me, I relearned words like "wonder" and "love" from her. And, more important, I learned how not to be embarrassed by simple sentiments.

Wonder.

One morning Holly woke me quite early, "Daddy, come quick! It's 'mazing!"

She led her grumpy dad to her bedroom.

"See!" She pointed. A huge full moon was setting in the west and through another window the sun, even larger was rising from the east at the same moment.

I sat with her on her bed and shared her awe.

Now and then I would stare at Holly in wonder. Her gentle face, her grace. Obviously God was a woman.

Then I would wonder at my wonder. Why didn't I spend every moment in amazement at her—at everybody?

Love.

With Holly no love was ever undemonstrated. Her good-night "I love you, Mommy, I love you, Daddy, was followed with hugs and kisses for all, especially the dog.

To Holly love was as real as a rock.

For Holly and her friends, affection was never muted. They didn't need a boozy cocktail party or a church moment of "peace" to inspire a kiss. Love was not just a word trotted out in a Sunday sermon and forgotten before the offering was taken. Their love for each other was a matter of every moment. To walk down the street holding hands or with their arms around each other wasn't a bit remarkable to them. Love was just the way it all was.

Because of Holly I could appreciate Tolstoy's "Confession"—"I believe in a God who is for me spirit, love, the principle of all things... I believe that the reason of life is for each of us simply to grow in love."

From Holly's instruction, I now could figure out what Meister Eckhart meant when he said, "If you love yourself you love everybody else as you do yourself. As long as you love another person less than you love yourself, you will not really succeed in loving yourself."

Of course, all this was a matter of faith—the faith that life is worth loving. That faith is "the force of life," as Tolstoy said.

It's all so simple and obvious, I thought. And it's not taught in church. People are complicated. God is simple. Love is God.

I covered my rocks with a blue tarp and headed south.

Weeks later the first snow buried everything.

III

{Mosquito Years}

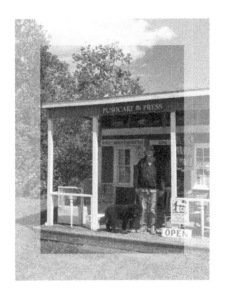

Down came the dry flakes, fat enough and heavy enough to crash like nickels on stone. It always surprised him, how quiet it was. Not like rain, but like a secret.

Toni Morrison

That January was one of the coldest months on recent record. Long Island Sound froze solid to Connecticut. Annie and I walked the shore and marveled at the stillness of the ice and snow-covered water, and the eerie silence. No waves, no tidal flow, no birds. The northeast was in lockdown.

In Maine the wind chill hit 100° below zero in 45 mile per hour gales. In nearby New Hampshire a park ranger, experienced in cold weather hiking, froze to death in his tent.

I imagined the broken-hearted cathedral foundation and our ring of rocks enduring the frigid brutality as they had for thousands of years, and would continue to do so for centuries more. After the cathedral toppled into ruins, a hunter or hiker might come upon the pile and realize somebody had attempted to build something here—a round something, certainly the circle indicated an impractical something. Perhaps an academic—if such still existed—would write a paper on it, a treatise on 21st century sun worship, a Druid revival, a burial pit. The academic wouldn't realize some of the rocks had names: "Holly," "Annie," and, I had decided, more local saints, with their stones.

On a whim I decided to head north into the

worst of it to check on the cathedral.

First Annie and I stopped in Amherst to visit Holly at Hampshire College. During the day, Lulu and I attempted to hike up a small nearby hill but the temperature, below zero, drove us back down. Although I didn't know it, Lulu, almost 10 years old, was in her last year, but gamely she attempted the hill in the finely powdered snow without complaint. At night we all huddled in the miniscule bedroom of our rental house while the temperature outside dropped below minus 20°.

School was out for the holidays in the five colleges of Amherst and Northampton but the place was never still. Far from the bucolic academic haven I had imagined, its malls swarmed with happy shoppers and its icy highways were clogged with motorists on missions of some sort. Overhead bombers from nearby Westfield airbase skimmed the clouds and announced regularly with their racket that a really big war was afoot in Iraq and we had a victory to accomplish. Between roaring bombers and racing cars, I wanted only out of the Pioneer valley and its Ivory Tower paradise.

Before I plunged North, we attended a shape note hymn recital at the Northampton Unitarian Church, a weekly event sponsored by the local Sacred Harp singers. For that evening, we were transported back 200 years to the earliest American hymn tradition of shape note singing.

No instruments, no microphones, no electronics of any sort. Only the leader's chopping hand and tapping shoe to keep the dozen singers together.

In that bitter chill, their singing was a primitive cry. None of the contemporary church musak. This stuff was deep in the gut. Sung with belief that did not doubt or compromise, that was not "nice", that poured from the anguish and hope of pioneers who had very little but their faith and a wilderness of uncertainty.

How could shopping malls, incessant traffic and omnipresent bombers have evolved from this great heart?

I hugged Holly and Annie goodbye the next day and, with shape note singers inspiring me, headed north for the cathedral site, hoping Lulu and I could find it in the snow.

Prayer

IT COULD BE THAT OUR FAITHLESSNESS IS A
COWERING COWARDICE BORN OF OUR VERY
SMALLNESS, A MASSIVE FAILURE OF IMAGI-
NATION... IF WE WERE TO JUDGE NATURE
BY COMMON SENSE OR LIKELIHOOD, WE
WOULDN'T BELIEVE THE WORLD EXISTED.

Annie Dillard

*A*fter an overnight stay at Brunswick, Maine's wonderfully seedy Siesta Motel, buried under plowed snow, Lulu and I arrived at icy Christy Hill and spun our car to the top.

Silence greeted us. (I've often thought of bottling Christy Hill silence. "Open the bottle and find peace.") And profound cold. The tower and the cabin, boarded up against snowdrifts, had survived the winter so far. None of the birches and beeches, snapped in the wind and ice, had crashed in their direction. Back in the woods, Lulu and I climbed through snow banks and over tree trunks to where I thought the broken hearted boulder was under the snow. Only the top of our rock pile gave it away. Footprints indicated that many animals had visited the site—deer, coyote, fox—but no boot marks from members of the Petroleum People—a race I imagine will enjoy tenure far shorter than other people in history. The PP have been around for barely 150 years and it seems not many of us will be left after the oil runs out. Will historians even know we were here at all? A junk car in a tar pit! But no PP had disturbed my sacred pile.

I blessed the rocks sleeping under the snow—each of them alive in their own atomic way. Some day they would all have the names of saints, I hoped. And in the spring they would be resurrected, blessed with mortar, and start their climb to the stars. It was too cold to attempt a stay in the cabin. A fire in the ancient Franklin stove would be of little help against the wind pouring over the Northeast hills. The sun was rapidly nearing its early January end. Lulu and I had to hit the road and find shelter. One could die up here.

At the foot of Christy Hill, Paul Sullivan had a small studio. I noticed his light was on, car outside. I drove a mile down the road, not wishing to stop and interrupt him. Then on impulse I turned around, drove back and knocked on his door. It sprang open. "Hendo!" he shouted, amazed that a summer person would show up in mid-winter, especially this mid-winter.

I apologized, said I was on my way back to Long Island, could only stay a minute and was told that a minute wouldn't do. I would be staying for dinner and the night at his home.

Paul, his wife Jill and young son Henry, lived not far away in an ancient colonial house, heated for the most part with a giant iron cooking stove. Jill had mastered that stove and prepared terrific meals burning logs from their ample wood pile.

Since the Sullivans owned no TV or other passive entertainment devices, Henry led off the evening with a reading from Ursula LeGuin's *Tales from*

Earthsea and Paul followed with a Bach Goldberg Variations selection on the living room's baby grand piano. In a few days he would be off to Japan to play for royalty with the Paul Winter group. He was amazed by all the advanced publicity reaching him from Japan: "Maybe they think we're the Beatles," he laughed.

At home, Paul volunteered for stints at the Penobscot Nursing home and earned his bread by teaching music at the Brooklin Elementary School and playing gigs at restaurants, halls and theaters up and down the Maine coast.

After Henry's reading and Paul's performance we settled around a small table near the giant stove. And Paul, from his South Boston Catholic memory, recited this prayer attributed to Saint Francis, which incredibly this Presbyterian boy had never heard before:

"Lord, make us instruments of your peace. Where there is hatred, let us sow love; where there is injury, pardon; where there is discord, union; where there is doubt, faith; where there is despair, hope; where there is darkness, light; where there is sadness, joy. Grant that we may not so much seek to be consoled as to console; to be understood as to understand; to be loved as to love. Amen."

In my suburban Philadelphia Protestant upbringing, we never prayed at table with such detailed fervor.

We raced through "Bless this food which we are about to eat and bless us to thy service" and please pass the mashed potatoes.

But Paul lingered after his recitation, then reached out to me and Henry and Jill and we quietly held hands, while Lulu and their hound Jemima snoozed at our feet.

The plea of the St. Francis prayer and the spirit surrounding our warm circle of hands were what I remembered the next day and long after as Lulu and I hurried south, over cold Maine highways.

There would be a stone in the cathedral for Paul and his family.

I DO NOT THINK IT IS IMPORTANT
WHETHER A MAN ENTERS RELIGION
BY THE FRONT DOOR OR THE BACK
DOOR, AS LONG AS HE ENTERS…
IF WE CAN ARRIVE AT A POSITION
IN WHICH JESUS ADMIRED THE
LILIES OF THE VALLEY AND ST.
FRANCIS LOVED THE BIRDS AS
GOD'S OWN CREATURES, WE HAVE
STUMBLED UPON THE VERY
SOURCE FROM WHICH ALL
RELIGIONS TOOK THEIR RISE.

Lin Yutang

t. Francis asked us to do the impossible: to offer love, forgiveness, faith, hope, light, and joy in place of hate, injury, doubt, despair, darkness and sadness.

He also hated cathedrals. This would become a useful architectural insight in the next few years.

For himself and his brothers he insisted on disposable huts.

It wasn't always that way for Francis. According to legend, after a misspent youth and a failed knighthood, Francis, son of a wealthy Assisi cloth merchant, received a message from God: "Francis, repair my house." He set about fixing up a deserted chapel in the forest. But he soon realized it wasn't the physical structure that needed repairing, it was the whole edifice of faith.

One day a visiting monk read him a Gospel passage. Jesus commanded "take no gold, nor silver, nor copper in your belt, no bag for your journey, nor two tunics, nor sandals nor a staff…and preach as you go saying, The Kingdom of Heaven is at hand."

Francis abandoned his chapel improvement project and cried out, "That's what I want. This is what I desire with all my soul!"

Francis fashioned a tunic out of rough cloth in the shape of a cross. His belt was rope, on his feet, nothing. His vow: "To follow the naked Christ."

His message—delivered to whomsoever he met—was simple. The three great evils are power, wealth, and knowledge (fancy academic learning). He was a primitive Christian, trying to walk in Christ's exact footprints. He cared not much for the Old Testament and everything for the New. To him, all that is required of us is a recognition of God's love and a constant meditation on that love. The ponderings of theologians are worthless.

Jesus owned nothing, neither should the brothers. Books, which were expensive, were banned, the Bible excepted. One might accumulate many books and pride oneself on a library, or on the false learning that books inspired.

Permanent housing was forbidden. His brothers should live in temporary reed shelters, or a cave would do, or a room donated from someone outside the flock. "If we owned anything we should have to have weapons to protect ourselves... we are resolved to own nothing temporal in this world."

For the final six years of his life, Francis fought being absorbed by the Church, a losing battle.

When a final rule for his new order was approved by the pope in 1223, it had gutted the founder's vision. Most of the Gospel passages were omitted, the language was dry, legalistic, and stripped of poetry. Gone were the admonitions to care for lepers, love poverty, and rebel against unworthy leaders.

Some possessions, books included, were permitted. Francis's paeans to the joy of manual labor were muted. The right to preach was now reserved for a few of the elect approved by bosses, not for all the brothers.

When he died on October 4, 1226, in agony, blind and covered with sores—some of them said to be stigmata from the crucified Christ—he was worshipped as a living saint. But by then he was more valued by the church for his relics—bits of hair, teeth, and bone—than for his continued living.

In short order his body was buried in a sumptuous basilica that would have shamed him.

It would be hard to justify my cathedral to St. Francis. So far this was no problem—just a circle of stones. Chartres would not have impressed St. Francis.

Perhaps a rock version of his reed hut would suffice.

HERE WE ARE, IN THE HOMELAND.
IT IS WINTER, AND IT WILL BE SPRING AGAIN.
WE HAVE KNOWN OTHER WINTERS, AND
SURVIVED THEM... I KNOW THESE TRUTHS.
LESSER TRUTHS WILL TAKE MORE LEARNING.

Hal Borland

{ SAINT ROCKS }

*R*ev. Rob McCall, in his deep winter Blue Hill Weekly Packet column, gave me some ideas for naming my cathedral saint rocks.

A friend pointed out that New York's St. John's cathedral, that imposing heap, had dedicated stones to poets and others, as has Westminster Abby in London and many others. I'd keep this tradition alive locally.

Rob reported:

"Being as how it is the middle of winter, let's mention some of the specimens of human nature that make life hereabouts absolutely incomparable. There's the formidable former state trooper and town constable who now and then puts on his leather jacket and bandanna to ride his motorcycle with his buddies, but also tenderly cares for his apple trees because he loves to "smell the beautiful blossoms." There's the burley, tooth-pick-chewing fire chief who is also an astounding artist and cartoonist, and carves delightful delicate decoys of local waterfowl. There's the past president of the proper ladies' garden club who trekked the entire Appalachian and Pacific Coast trails, certainly no bed of roses. There's the local dentist who can make you laugh 'til you cry even with a mouthful of cotton wads, and plays the hottest 5-string banjo you've ever heard. There's the ER physician's assistant who can give a quick tracheotomy with a ball point pen, if necessary to save your life; and then sing you some rocking gospel with piano or bluegrass bass, if necessary to save your soul. There's the dedicated EMT who is also a Magus of Magic. There's the town meeting moderator who just happens to be Buddhist and an acupuncturist. There's the local elementary school music teacher who has just won a Grammy. There's the artist who can paint pictures and sing songs that will make your hair stand on end, is married to a preacher, and has a dress of Emmy Lou Harris's hanging in her closet. There are countless able carpenters with degrees in philosophy and religion and English and sociology [all of which come in mighty handy on certain jobs]. There are scores of amazing artists who create works of surpassing beauty while their kids are off to school. There are dozens of steel drum players who bring the sweet sounds of the warm West Indies to the cold coast of Maine. Honestly, this is just scratching the surface: these marvels go on and on all around our little towns."

In my journal I added Rob's suggestions to my list of saint rocks.

Churches

OH, WARM LIGHT, COULDN'T YOU HAVE WAITED A LITTLE LONGER? HOW SAFE WE WERE IN THE DEAD OF WINTER, HOW GENTLY WE DREAMED. HOW BEAUTIFUL IT WAS TO SLEEP UNDER THE SNOW!

Kate Barnes

{ CHURCHES }

For two decades, by Holly's birthday on March 14, the crocuses on Long Island had bloomed. Not this year. The early shoots barely peeked above the frozen ground. It was April before the crocuses were in full flower, scattered across the lawn in whites and purples.

That hard winter evolved into a slog of a spring. I was, as usual out of shape and pounds heavier in body and spirit. With some reluctance I had accepted a second term on the Session of the Presbyterian church down the road. I loved the spirit of the few dozen or so regular members, but they could be a contentious lot and it was always hard keeping the church united and the bills paid.

Ministers came and went.

We were too tiny for their ambitions. Bigger and richer congregations beckoned.

The Irish minister who had welcomed me back to the faith years before with his humor and energy and ready doubts about doctrine, had been defrocked by the Long Island Presbytery for dallying with a woman who was not his soon-to-be-ex-wife. His detractors in the congregation had gone to the trouble of lurking in his girlfriend's shrubbery with a video camera to catch him messing about.

The tape was rather damning—the pastor walking about in a bathrobe—and out he went.

Another preacher, a large fellow, much too fat for the pulpit, longed to be loved by the congregation but wasn't. He accused them of being "clergy killers"—and out he too went.

Our present pastor, the best so far, was a woman of great energy and charm, a temporary "supply" replacement. She had inducted me as an Elder as I kneeled on the floor in front of her and the congregation.

Our little church persevered through all its battles and I did what I could to help, a lesson reading at services now and then, advice on housekeeping matters (snow plowing, cleaning, wages, etc.) at Session meetings. But it was a roilsome lot, split down the middle into camps. Church attendance there was often bad for my spiritual health. For months I stayed away.

In fact "organized religion," an awful but accurate label, is usually not conducive to an exalted spirituality. The "frozen chosen" is a cliché with teeth. Such a frost is what I'd seek to avoid in the Maine woods, an antidote to a childhood of picky admonitions and an overshadowing terror of hell, plus a steady dose of friendly pastors with ghastly messages of imminent doom. I am happy to say those messages have gradually evolved over my life into a love proclamation, with hell seldom whispered. Unlike the church of my childhood, love has won, at least for now and for the congregations I find myself in.

Back then, my good, shy and rigidly orthodox dad drove his family to the church of his own Philadelphia childhood—Oak Park Fourth Presbyterian. We kids were regaled with all the usual Old Testament tales of the Diety's genocide, plus mass slaughter by God's victorious armies and assurances that we were on the right side if only we believed in Jesus, memorized our Bible verses, and attended Sunday School without fail. These were handy guarantees in the era of Nazis, Communists and the atomic Armageddon. My brother and my sister and I loved and trusted our gentle parents and we did not, dared not, ask questions.

Later, as I hit puberty, we moved into the Main Line suburbs and joined the upscale Bryn Mawr Presbyterian Church, an edifice with an imposing steeple that sought to prove it had the right stuff for its solid and wealthy congregation sheltering under its copper roof. The white-haired minister was named Rex Clements. In the balcony next to Rex Clements's American flag bedecked altar were the permanent pews of Allen Dulles, head of the CIA, and the head of International Telephone and Telegraph and other powers.

The very least of these powers was my kind father in his only Sunday suit, who couldn't imagine himself in any sort of lofty pew, except that bestowed by the grace of Jesus. I knew he felt crushed by that huge building and those eminent operators. He parked his ancient Chevy on a side street out of sight of the Rolls Royces lined up in the church driveway with chauffeurs polishing the chrome.

Summers in Ocean City, New Jersey, we worshipped in less pompous circumstances—at a wooden "Tabernacle" on Sunday and a tiny beach side chapel for Wednesday night hymn sings. In both ecumenical gatherings my father was at home, and much later, in similar ocean churches, I too would feel something genuine again where Christ wasn't mocked by chrome-polishing chauffeurs.

He delivered his 'news right fresh from heaven' by reading the Beatitudes... Then at seventy-two years of age, forty-six devoted to his self-imposed mission, he ripened into death as naturally and beautifully as the seeds of his own planting had grown into bud and blossom and fruit.

Harper's Magazine
on the death of Johnny Appleseed, 1847

{A MODEST PROPOSAL}

*A*pple trees by the dozens grow on the land surrounding my hilltop, untended, utterly forgotten, some perhaps planted by Johnny Appleseed. Deep in the woods I found trees that were obviously part of a long gone homestead. The earth was ringed with rotten apples, those the deer and bears had rejected.

In the spring of the cathedral's next year, I came upon a young bear, his head resting against an apple tree, down a steep slope by a dirt road. Lulu and I had set off to the general store and Lulu stopped to pee—an occupation I find helpful for observations—man or beast. Peeing forces you to concentrate your gaze for a few moments. I saw the bear at rest, asleep I thought, as if sleeping off a fermented apple bender. But he never stirred. For a week he rested there, hit by a car the game warden said later. Soon the stench of his decomposing made the village roads people haul him off to the county landfill.

The death of the young bear was a bad start to that spring, already poisoned by Bush's phony Iraq war. Our Christian president ("Jesus changed my life") had declared "shock and awe" on the people of Baghdad. We got to see his sacred war live on TV, thousands of innocents ("collateral damage") slaughtered in massive explosions, like a Fourth of July extravaganza. I and much of the world had protested Bush's oil-mad extermination. It was hopeless. We had no say. The administration faked its way into made-for-TV entertainment with imbedded reporters chattering their way through the desert in tank bellies.

By now this unspeakable fraud is old news, but I wondered then, and still do, how is it that we roast people as if at a suburban barbeque? What a waste of good meat. After Jonathan Swift's "A Modest Proposal" I composed a screed on the economic wisdom of cannibalism. Why waste all this tender flesh? Harvest it from corpses and can it. If human consumption of humans turns you off, pack it for pigs.

My screed went into the desk drawer. Who would publish such an idea, even if it did make perfect money-saving sense.

Early April in Maine was no balm to my spirit. While the rest of the country marveled at daffodils and tulips, villagers hungered for the slightest hint of green. Mounds of snow hid my wood pile when Lulu and I arrived to open up the cabin. There was no hope of mortaring cathedral stone until June so all we could do was sit by the saints rock pile and wonder what would bring back hope.

Worse news was that my friends Doris Grumbach and Sybil Pike, who ran a unique antiquarian bookstore nearby, decided they had become too old for Maine winters. Next fall they were moving from their cove-side home to an assisted care facility in eastern Pennsylvania. I was losing the companionship and warm hearth of two good friends.

Doris, in her late eighties, a novelist and book critic, continued to write exquisite memoirs about the simple joys and rigors of advancing age, while Sybil tended rare volumes at Wayward Books. But Maine had defeated them.

I wondered, sitting on that pile, if it would finally defeat me too. Lulu looked up at me, her gaze as always steadfast. "What's next?" she seemed to ask. We walked off into the snow to split some logs for the Franklin stove. A blizzard was still possible this time of year.

I WISH, O SON OF THE LIVING GOD, O ANCIENT, ETERNAL KING, FOR A HIDDEN LITTLE HUT IN THE WILDERNESS THAT IT MAY BE MY DWELLING... FRAGRANT LEEK, HENS, SPECKLED SALMON, TROUT, BEES. RAIMENT AND FOOD ENOUGH FOR ME FROM THE KING OF FAIR FAME, AND I TO BE SITTING FOR A WHILE PRAYING GOD IN EVERY PLACE.

9th century Irish

Hermit's Song

*L*ulu and I slept in the tower that first night, me under piles of blankets. From the tower the sunrise over Mt. Desert Island and the ocean would be spectacular.

About 4:30 a.m. I held my hand in front of my face, my test for first light. But I couldn't see it. A half hour later I thought I saw the outline of my fingers and fifteen minutes later it was so—the light was coming. Not long after I made out Lulu at the foot of the bed, and she raised her head: breakfast yet?

We listened to the silence.

Then gradually over the mountain a pale glow and the bare trees in silhouette and the first bird—a tentative song.

And the silence again.

I buried deeper under the covers. The temperature said 28°. Until that sun hit the tower I wasn't moving.

Then another bird, and soon the whole springtime choir. It was time to sing out and no right-minded bird would be caught songless.

Soon the red squirrels began their perpetual chattering complaints with the world, including the squirrel who had declared the cabin his very own and wanted us gone from the premises. He was escorted out hanging on the end of a broom later in the morning, chattering bitterly. He stole Lulu's kibble from her bowl for days until retiring to the woodpile for the spring.

The sun rose over Mt. Desert, hit the tower, and up to the tower's peak I climbed to watch the silver shining move over the ocean, illuminating the patch between Gott and Placentia islands.

There were spring chores to do—clean the oven and drawers of mouse turds first. But there were few turds—thanks to Rob McCall's "Bounce" instructions. Sheets of Bounce fabric softener worked in his Eastport camp and it worked here too. Mice hate "Spring fragrance" it turns out and flee at the mere whiff of Bounce sheets distributed throughout the cabin.

I turned on the gas and made coffee and fed Lulu and off we went down the western blueberry field to meet our new neighbors Jeff Buchhotz and his wife Michele and their Labrador puppy Jack. They had bought an old house that needed just about everything. Jeff was getting started evenings and weekends on repairs while not working as a welder at Brooklin Boatyard, and nurturing his own home business, Sputnik Tools, which made gadgets for bicycle repairs.

Jeff's was one of many cottage enterprises in the neighborhood. Pete Douvarjo, my neighbor on the right, was a certified backwoods Maine Guide. Up the dirt road was Chuck Marshall, one of the finest carpenters on the peninsula.

Later that summer Pushcart would open a book-store next to the Sedgwick Antiques in a 10 x 14 shed, the "World's Smallest Bookstore" I claimed, although I never really checked the rest of the world too closely.

Back from a visit with Jeff and Michele, Lulu and I stopped to talk with Ron Salman. An MIT dropout, he had lived on this hill since the early 70's in a converted chicken barn. His lettuce was already planted and he gave me lessons on making compost and what to plant and when.

Since I was starting with rocky shallow soil I needed raised beds filled with useful dirt. The lumber for the beds was donated by Maine Guide Pete—his daughter had left for college and the lumber from her old tree house became my garden borders.

For soil I mucked out Paul Sullivan's sheep pens and what his three sheep didn't provide I augmented with tubs of goat manure from nearby Sunset Farms, where a dozen goats stood around me nibbling at the Volvo's trim and windshield wiper, staring at me like they knew something profound that I was too dumb to figure out.

Soon my beds were filled with rich muck and the first seeds planted and spring was really coming on fast. The green would rise suddenly and right after-ward the weeds would begin their mighty, inevitable attack.

Just outside of Ellsworth, John Blogett from his garage ran the Love Barn, named for what I never figured out. He dealt not in love but in marvelous ancient stoves, including some kitchen behemoths that were decked out in trim like a 1950s Buick. From John I bought a modest glass fronted used Waterford for $120, delivered. The airtight Waterford would provide serious heat, that my Franklin Stove lacked. Blizzard proofing. John helped me install it.

Near the Love Barn, Bryan Emlen ran Choice Auto Repair from his home. He patched up my rock hauling clunker when necessary. Chickens roosted on the car roof as Bryan worked. His young daughter sat on the porch steps and shooed off the chickens when they interfered with dad's job.

These people had all survived the brutal winter in good health and strong spirits and with a warming welcome for this fellow and his mongrel dog from away, who obviously needed all the help and advice and warmth he could get.

And finally, later in the season, the great event— the Bee Man returned to our blueberry fields, his truck filled with hives. The bees would pollinate the next blueberry crop, if the bears didn't devour their hives first.

Only then did I regain faith that these fields were safe from the developers who were planning subdivisions, condos and cell phone towers all over coastal Maine. The Bee Man's arrival meant that the Petroleum People had not yet taken over. For now, at least, the bears and the blueberries had it.

The spring was unfolding beautifully. Even the black flies had been late in arriving, but soon I knew they too would emerge from the deep chill.

I was falling in love with Christy Hill all over again—especially its waving people. Walkers, drivers, joggers, bikers—they all waved to me. I was reminded of Holly, as a child, waving and waving. Hello, hello, whoever you are. No introduction needed.

By mid-May it was still too cold to mortar stones, so Lulu and I headed off into the deep woods to visit various ponds and streams, wary of mama bears recently out of their winter dens, hungry and out of sorts, often with cubs to protect from the likes of us. I sang and whistled as I hiked to warn the mamas—"Whistle while you work"—while Lulu plowed ahead in her own rapture determined to discover the next great sniff.

Soon it would be warm enough to begin again with the mortar and saint stones.

THE YOUTH GETS TOGETHER HIS MATERIALS
TO BUILD A BRIDGE TO THE MOON...
OR PERCHANCE A PALACE OR TEMPLE ON
EARTH, AND AT LENGTH THE MIDDLE AGED
MAN CONCLUDES TO BUILD A WOODSHED
WITH THEM.

Thoreau

*D*uring my years in Maine I have come to expect a reasonable progression of seasons: cool and wet in May and June, hot in July, dry and warm in August, chilly and bright in September and October. But this summer broke all the rules. In June it seldom rose above 50°; in mid-July, when 80° was a high norm, we hit 41° and stayed in a chill until the end of September.

Any thought of mortaring rocks was out of the question. I busied about the site cutting back dead beech trees and brush for the cathedral that might some day rise there.

I could work chopping trees and brush because it required constant motion. If I stopped briefly, the black flies and mosquitoes were on me immediately. One of my theories of Maine workers' moving so adroitly and snappily is that constant motion keeps the bugs from settling. Hard, quick work is a great bug repellant. Most repellants wear off quickly. Not work.

To select, contemplate and place rocks was impossible, even if the chill would let mortar harden. Just lifting a rock into position invited bug bites, and to sit and ponder shapes and joinings and plumb was to invite insect oblivion.

Black flies arrived early in May as fog banks rolled in from the sea, and stayed for days. All night fog accumulated on the leaves and dripped like a steady rain. The black flies enjoyed this weather. It lubricated their mating.

A black fly bite is unlike that of a bee or mosquito. Black flies don't sting, they chew. As tiny as pin heads, they burrow unnoticed under hat band, collar, sleeves or socks and munch away, leaving welts that itch for days and in some people produce illness and fatal reactions. Farther north herds of caribou are driven mad by swarms of chewing black flies. In blind, hopeless panic they race across the tundra seeking and not finding escape.

In Sedgwick people clamped on helmets with screens that fell over their heads and necks and resembled the armor of medieval knights. That summer many such knights hiked the roads and woods, anonymous behind their bug gear. But it was annoying to build with such decoration, even if the weather had been warm enough and the almost daily rain didn't promise to wipe out fresh mortar.

In the cold drizzle and fog drip Lulu and I couldn't romp through the wet fields with any joy. Most days Lulu hid under the cabin porch, as depressed as I was by the constant gloom.

Indoors, I attempted to finish a book about the hymns of my life that I had been writing for five years, a personal hymnal. But most days the music and words lay on a damp and unenthusiastic page. "Simple Gifts" I would call the book later.

I tried prayer, but forgot what I was praying to. As George Bernanos reminded me in *Diary of a Country Priest*, "If you can't pray, at least say your prayers." I forgot that too.

In June, as the black flies died off, the mosquitoes attacked, fresh from cool puddles. Well into fall the swarms never diminished. Some evenings mosquitoes were lined up 30 to 40 a screen as the visiting Annie and Holly escaped them on the porch. And of course one or two always made it into the cabin and whined all night, keeping us awake while we itched the last of our abysmal black fly welts.

The garden was drowning. A first crop of carrots and lettuce went under; a second crop of kale, soybeans, yellow snap beans and tomatoes was mired in wet goat and sheep crap. When the cabbage did get close to harvest, an army of slugs finished it off in a day. A slug is a mysterious being. In dry weather it is not to be seen; in rain it suddenly and miraculously appears crawling out of the dust and laying waste to what it wills.

Our flowers—morning glories, day lilies, rudbeckia, honeysuckle, wild iris, lupine, petunia and impatiens did better—until beetles did some of them in.

The gardens were an act of faith. We could have purchased most of the vegetables at the local farmers markets for a much cheaper price than growing them. But garden rebirth was important to me and my neighbors. Life was renewed. Especially in that awful era of "Shock and Awe," a garden was a spiritual necessity. A garden kept us hopeful, if not sane.

I turned to the Pushcart bookstore. Every morning I'd bike down Christy Hill, with Lulu close behind, open the "World's Smallest Bookstore," and talk to visitors on the porch. In each other we found a sort of salvation in that summerless summer.

THE OLD PEOPLE CAME TO LOVE THE SOIL
AND SAT OR RECLINED ON THE GROUND WITH
A FEELING OF BEING CLOSE TO A MOTHERING
POWER... THAT IS WHY THE OLD INDIAN
STILL SITS UPON THE EARTH TO COME CLOSER
IN KINSHIP TO OTHER LIVES AROUND.

Luther Standing Bear

The Pushcart Bookstore may (or may not) be the world's smallest bookstore—but it is certainly the only bookstore with a porch as big as the store itself. On that porch, festooned with yard sale rocking chairs and a beat up wicker couch, I greeted my neighbors.

Pushcart had gained a minor celebrity for the memoir I'd written about building the tower, published by Farrar Straus and Giroux a few years earlier. Tourists stopped on the road and peeped through the bushes at me. They took pictures. "See that's the guy!" I was a combination of hero and oddball. I mean who erects a wooden tower on a windy hill without knowing what he is doing and confesses his foolishness. "That guy—see!"

I didn't enjoy the tourists. I felt like a caged zoo animal. But at the World's Smallest Bookstore I met my neighbors, previously unknown to me, who lived deep in the woods down lonely dirt roads. Local people were unimpressed with celebrity.

Sitting on that porch was like a seat at Thornton Wilder's "Our Town." All of Sedgwick and much of the peninsula drove or walked past at least once a day and many stopped to talk, or maybe even buy a book.

Charlie Smith, who stood at about 5'6", was a World War II B52 tailgunner who flew missions deep into Germany before being shot down and rescued. At war's end he was hired as a pilot for the Rockefeller family and was a lode of information about the peculiarities of Nelson, David, and the rest of the Rockefellers. Now nearly 90 he mourned his wife of 60 years, Polly, dead from ovarian cancer.

Charlie was waging a one man campaign against the doctor who misdiagnosed Polly's disease, and the entire Maine board of doctor certification. Singlehandedly Charlie had unearthed documents on half a dozen doctors who had gained licenses while previously convicted of personal misrepresentation and outright crimes. He charged into the powerful medical fraternity like a tiny, elderly Don Quixote and managed to shake up state politicians and doctors both. Charlie got the rules changed, and many lives were saved by "Old Charlie" as he called himself.

Later, when I was enduring cancer treatments, Charlie turned up at the cabin with a huge weed whacker and trimmed my field when I couldn't. Old age was not about to stop old Charlie.

A saint rock for him.

Alice Hildebrand didn't come to the church via a strict religious upbringing (like myself) or a flash of salesmanship at a tent revival. Alice lived a hard life and ended up somehow as the beloved minister of the First Congregational Church of Deer Isle.

When she visited me on the store porch one rainy morning, she was not yet ordained, but as leader of a Bible study class she taught me much about the religion I thought I knew—about ever evolving ideas of God, the changing lens that each generation sees through. At her class we read Marcus Borg's wonderful *Reading the Bible Again for the First Time* and we were not afraid to attack the very church we belonged to —me as a Presbyterian elder and Alice as a 40 plus year old minister in training. Nothing was sacred to us because everything was sacred.

Alice, an active member of Alcoholics Anonymous, was not coy about her past. She had suffered from various addictions—booze, pills, meth (meth was the hardest to beat she said). For years she had sampled other callings, as a Quaker, as a Pentacostalist, as nothing at all.

She had always lived on the peninsula, getting by as a waitress, a blueberry raker, and anything else that came up. She once spent a frigid winter as a single mom with her young son, in the ancient, uninsulated Sedgwick Customs House.

Somehow she found her way to the Congregational Church and a faith born from suffering and doubt. She married Allen Myers, a professor of geology, who had made his own way from rocks to later ordination as minister in the Brooksville Congregational Church, perhaps the loveliest church in all of Maine, with a steeple twice as high as the structure beneath it, and a dwindling congregation. Allen, who was a ten year survivor of tonsil cancer ("sure to kill you in six years," said his doctor) made it his mission to save that church, but with an aging membership and only a few children attending, it would be hard. When such churches died, the summer people snapped them up for quaint vacation habitats.

One day Alice and Allen visited my cathedral site. We sat briefly on the broken-hearted boulder.

Allen informed me that what I had here was a ledge of Sedgwick Pluton (granite to me). The stones were gneiss (looks like granite but is crumbly), Ellsworth schist (greenish and thinly layered), Oak Point granite (zoned crystals, whatever that was) and sandstone.

All these rocks had endured through endless time to be named by Professor/Reverend Myers for me. He and Alice had traveled their own hardscrabble trails to find each other.

Alice and Allen both get saint rocks—a pretty, greenish Ellsworth schist.

Dud Hendrick dropped by the porch. I knew him from his Pilgrim Inn days. He and his wife Jean owned the inn and traded me glasses of red wine for recent Pushcart titles. I masqueraded as a backwoods Mainer to entertain his guests. But that was long ago.

Now Dud was just back from a bike ride from Ho Chi Minh City to Saigon, a reconciliation tour, American soldiers and their former Vietnamese enemies, together, forgiving.

Dud was a graduate of the U.S. Naval Academy where he was an all-American lacrosse star in the 60's. He volunteered for service in Vietnam, a demolition expert. He disassembled Viet Cong and North Vietnam bombs before they killed, and he knew how to build one too. Then, gradually, the war turned his stomach. He saw what it did to his comrades and how it devastated Vietnamese and Cambodian civilians by the hundreds of thousands. Out of uniform he began his mission against the perpetual American war machine.

When Bush invaded Iraq, Dud and others mobilized the Peninsula Peace and Justice Committee. In all seasons, Dud and others stood protest witness by the roadsides of peninsula towns. They waved peace flags and "Out of Iraq" banners. "Honk if you agree" one sign asked. In early days, few drivers honked. A flip of the middle finger or curses were the response. But Dud and company never quit their weekly demonstrations and finally there were more honks than curses.

That summer I sometimes joined Dud by the Deer Isle main street. In the house behind our small demonstration lived the father of a boy who was fighting in Iraq. He hated us, figured we were accusing his son of a crime. He screamed violent profanities at our backs and cranked up his stereo with patriotic marches at top volume.

Dud tried to calm him down, talking to him as a veteran, not a commie pinko. But the fellow was psychotic with rage. Any minute I thought we might be shot in the back.

But it never happened. Throughout the years of the Iraq war Dud and his Peace and Justice Committee stood their ground. The curses subsided, the patriotic stereo was turned off, the honks were 100%.

For his bike ride through postwar Vietnam with former enemy soldiers—featured in an ABC TV documentary—for his persistence against Bush and Cheney's atrocities, Dud gets a saint stone. Although, as an agnostic, I doubt if he wants one.

THERE HAVE ALWAYS BEEN THOSE WHO LOVED [THE WEATHER] FOR ITS OWN SAKE... THEY DELIGHT IN EXTREMES. THEY ARE GRATEFULLY AWARE THAT NOBODY CAN REGULATE THE WEATHER, NOR CHARGE ADMISSION TO IT, AND ARE HAPPY THAT IT IS FOREVER OUT OF THE REACH OF POLITICIANS.

T. M. Longstreth

And so the non-summer passed and suddenly everybody was leaving.

Doris and Sybil closed Wayward Books for good, packed up for the Pennsylvania assisted living village, and donated some of their books to Pushcart's store.

Holly, who had stayed through most of that awful summer working as a gardener, left for a junior semester in Barcelona, and Annie headed back to Long Island and her duties as head of the local public access TV station.

Before they left I mixed up some mortar in hot stove water and we set a rock in the cathedral in honor of our family, a lovely, gray Henderson stone. I scrubbed it with the wire brush and settled it into a bed of warm mortar on the altar. If the temperature remained above 50° for a bit, it might actually stay there.

Then they were gone. Just Lulu and me, expecting only more cold and rain, as the sun set farther to the south and the dark night increased quickly.

I was almost finished with the book about hymns, or it had finished me. I was wading through a massive draft of essays about the hymns I loved with no way to organize it all.

Then suddenly it was summer. The winds picked up from the south, the constant rain and fog lifted and it was t-shirt weather in the bugless woods. Summer in October.

Lulu and I got busy at the rock pile on each blessed, freakish day—temperature in the 70's by day and 50's by night.

In two weeks I completed four circles of the cathedral wall. We were on a swift upward quest to wherever it was we were questing.

A visitor, if I had any, might see a real edifice arising here in the gold and orange woods. Soon my problem would be how to widen the wall so it wouldn't topple over as it rose, a double wall.

This was going to work! In my journal I wrote "I come alive again after a busy, buggy, rain-sodden summer wondering where my soul had gone. I start to *see* again!"

It was time for a minor celebration at the Brooklin pub. Since I had no shower except for a plastic bag warmed in the weak sun—useless now—I visited Paul Sullivan's house to shower off the day's mortar dust. The afternoon sunlight from a small bathroom window crossed my chest.

In any other angle of light I wouldn't have seen the horror there, the valleys and ridges on my left breast. It was lumpy, pockmarked and the nipple was indented. A strange yellow ugliness permeated the skin, and underneath it something was growing.

A muscle maybe. But no muscle belonged there.

A monster was clawing at me, as quietly as a black fly chewed.

I tried not to believe what this meant.

My sister had breast cancer at 36, and beat it. My mother died of breast cancer after a twelve year struggle.

But men didn't get breast cancer did they? A trip to the Blue Hill Library and a medical guide revealed that indeed they did, not usually, but male breast cancer wasn't that rare either. The encyclopedia described a treatment: the testicles were sliced off to reduce testosterone and estrogen, the two hormones who danced with each other in male and female.

"10/24/04 Definite lump in breast, nipple indented—bk almost finished—will do—then leave," I scribbled in my journal.

I locked up the bookstore, the tower and the cabin, wrapped the cathedral walls in blue tarps against the winter and fled with Lulu and the draft of my hymn book.

I'd need every song in that book in the years ahead, if I could remember the words, and if I could sing at all.

IV
{Cancer Years}

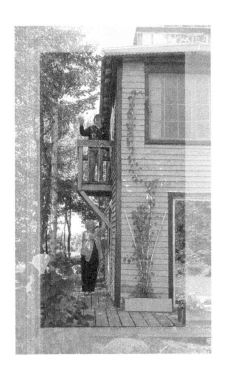

Biopsy

"CLOUDS COME FROM TIME TO TIME—
AND BRING A CHANCE TO REST FROM LOOKING AT
THE MOON."

Bashō

*C*astration? I couldn't whisk these visions away with any hymn I knew—"There is a Balm in Gilead," "Abide With Me." Forget it.

I was caught between despair and the name of Jesus. That is all that remained of my faith. One word. No song. No hymn. A friend who had been to horror and back. Jesus.

As the ferry took Lulu and me across Long Island Sound, I was far from thoughts of cathedrals, from sun, moon, stars, seas and golden fall. I was entering technoland—plastic, stainless steel, florescent light. Blake Kerr, my doctor sat me on a table and palpitated the yellow lump. "It could be anything" he said and ordered a mammogram.

The Breast Health room of the local hospital was done up in pink. I sat in the small waiting room with two anxious women, who stared at me, questioning why I was there at all. This was the Ladies Room and I was perhaps misinformed. Certainly I was out of place.

My name was called and I was ushered into a chamber by a nurse who was captain of a large machine. No prayer this, no wishful thinking, no glad singing. This was the facts. A cold gadget was clamped on the limited flesh of my left breast. From another room, the nurse flipped some switches, paused and emerged to tell me she'd have to consult with a doctor "in case we need more images."

Shivering, I sat in a chair in my gown and paged through an old *Family Circle* magazine. The door opened. Somebody walked in. I looked up. The door slammed behind him. The doctor. Grim. "I'm afraid these images are worrisome. We'll need a biopsy," Dr. Glück announced.

"When?" I asked.

The door slammed again behind him, the same awful finality. It opened. "They can see you now" and he gave me a room number.

Two guys and another machine. I was laid out on a table, they injected my left breast with novocaine and prepared their sonogram and needle probe.

Suddenly I was scared, not for me but for Lulu, who waited in the car parked on a side street. My father had died suddenly of a heart attack. What if this needle was more than my heart could stand. What if I died right here? Nobody would know that Lulu was in that parked car.

So I explained it all to the two guys, which street she was on and how I might die and she'd die because nobody knew where she was. They nodded and figured I was a bit strange, I guess. A dog is my major worry in a crisis like this? A dog?

And they got to work. The novocaine was useless. I felt stabbed and said so.

"More novocaine?"

"Please."

The pain was amazing.

The guys and I watched the sonogram image. A long, ragged snake sucked its way from the inverted nipple outward. It had no purpose. No goal. No form. It meant merely to advance, wherever it wandered. Mindless.

"That's cancer" I said.

They didn't disagree, jabbing me again from another angle into the snake.

I made it to the car. Lulu, who as ever was joy itself on my return, insisted that I be glad too. I tried.

The next day, cold, raining, at noon, Dr. Glück called. "Sorry, it's cancer."

IT GETS DARKER AND DARKER,
THEN JESUS COMES.

Wendell Berry

{A Visit}

And then love happened.

From people I'd forgotten, from saint stone neighbors and neighbors I barely knew, from friends I'd ignored or seldom seen, love poured forth. This then was the hymn that followed me from the cathedral.

One morning before my surgery, Lulu slept on the floor. I lay on the sunroom couch, tired, weak, apprehensive. Paul Sullivan telephoned from Maine to wish me well and said that Reverend McCall had mentioned my name on the Sunday prayer list at the Blue Hill Congo.

After we said good-bye the room filled with what I can only describe as a force, as if the air pressure had tripled. It wasn't a vision of light and love, but a sensation of universal power. I skeptically tried to explain it away as a mood of the moment brought on by the phone call from Maine but couldn't, and although I expected it to fade away immediately— and begged it not to—the presence lingered with me and Lulu for perhaps half an hour before gradually leaving.

It is easy to dismiss such accounts. We have read endless tales of Jesus and Mary or a saint appearing to true believers in a pizza pie crust or a wallpaper stain. But I cannot deny that force. It was unexpected and not requested. I needed comfort and assurance, not force. But force I got. Nothing gentle about it.

One of the most convincing visitations from the Thin Places in all of literature is that of the late novelist Reynolds Price in his classic memoir of cancer recovery, *A Whole New Life*. Price's cancer, unlike mine, was exceedingly painful, a tumor that curled down his spine, also like a snake. He endured months of radiation therapy.

One morning, Price says, he fell into an exhausted sleep. He was transported to the shores of the Sea of Galilee. Jesus came toward him. Price called out to him about his pain, and chances for survival. Jesus said merely "Your sins are forgiven," and turned and walked away. Price complained to himself that his sins were not exactly what bothered him at the moment. He asked Jesus about ending the pain, and would he live? Jesus said simply—"That too." And Price found himself back in his room.

He did indeed survive, for many years confined to a wheelchair. And he learned to manage the pain.

Price is quick to criticize his memory of this event. As a respected literary critic, he wouldn't accept this as a piece of Hallmark sentimentality. Perhaps his pain had driven him over the edge? No, he answers, this visit was real. Jesus did speak those

six words. Not a vision, not a metaphor, not wishful thinking, not temporary insanity. No question.
Real.

In the same way, I cannot question the force in
my room—St. Francis, Jesus, The Holy Spirit, none
of the above—it makes no difference. Something
else had been with my dog and me that afternoon. I
long for it to return.

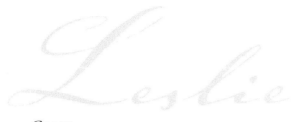

Grace—
TO BE ACCEPTED BY THAT WHICH IS
GREATER THAN YOU.

Paul Tillich

𝒟r. Leslie Lopez Montgomery swept into her office deep underground at Memorial Sloan-Kettering Hospital in New York—coiffed brunette hair, non-sensible shoes, a stunning can-do lady.

She shook hands with Annie and me and I presented her with a recent Pushcart Prize edition. I wanted her to know I wasn't just another patient, not a number—as if a male breast cancer case wasn't distinction enough. She took the book, thanked me, plopped it down on a chair.

She did some basic feeling of lymph nodes and tumor then penciled an outline how she'd cut it all out. A machine would do my breathing for me for two plus hours. A machine! I'd have none of it. Ignoring me, Leslie headed down the hall to her computer—"How's next Thursday sound to you?" she called, as if it were a lunch date.

Days later, after many pre-surgery tests, Annie and I walked forty blocks to Sloan-Kettering on Manhattan's Upper East Side holding hands. It was a stunning November day; fall had finally drifted down from Maine to New York. For a while we sat in a park near the hospital. Children on recess raced around us shouting and laughing in the falling leaves. To calm myself I repeated my friend Pat

Strachan's advice—she had endured a colon cancer operation years before—"Just let them take care of you."

I checked in at the hospital and was greeted by unfailingly kind nurses, given a gown, and I walked into the operating room where Leslie, who in her youth, beauty, and thoughtfulness reminded me of my daughter, (I told her so), talked with me as her team did various things to my body. I went under laughing at the color-splattered cap of one assistant. "That's ridiculous," were my final words.

When I woke up in recovery, missing a left breast and some chest hair, Leslie was bending over me: "Your lymph nodes are clean, Mr. Henderson. Your prognosis is good."

"Hot shit! I blurted, rather inappropriately.

The next two days were a storm of love.

Holly called from her semester of studies in Barcelona. She later wrote that she lit a candle for me in a small church by the Mediterranean shore. "Dad, I sat in the church for a little while, staring at the candle and listening to the private service for a family member who had passed away. For the candle I chose one of the many saints that spoke to me. The statue was of a man on his side, sleeping peacefully, with his shirt open, baring his chest. Two seashells covered each breast. It meant a lot to me."

In my semi-private room, just to the other side of a curtain that divided us, a young man, Mark

Harris, spent the night sleepless and throwing up, a stomach tumor. The next day, Mark's friends visited him and read Bible selections and prayed. Now and then, Mark and I talked over the curtain and in the night I silently tried to send him some of the force of the presence that had visited me days before.

The idea of death became very real in that room, but so did the love that Annie, friends, doctors, and nurses brought to me and Mark. As Emily Dickinson wrote: "That love is all there is/Is all I know of love."

Love was all I had there. Ego was obliterated. "Self" seemed silly, a pasted-together mirage. The real was exactly what St. Francis said it is: "In the giving of ourselves we receive, and in dying we're born to eternal life."

Faith I didn't know I had, from my childhood, bred in the bone, carried me through those days and the long, often confusing and depressing years of consultations and treatment that followed.

Since I realized that "I" didn't even exist to start with, death became meaningless. "I" was free. We are all free.

Journal entry

"10:20 am/porch/EH/Tue/11/23/04/Sun

"I'm on the other side of the op/2draining tubes and bulbs attached to ace bandage—big incision from breast bone to arm pit (left side)—no

pain/no pills/never was much pain/got mor-
phine in IV drip, removed next day/back home
next afternoon...Having looked at death up close
and anticipating a return engagement, I am in no
mood to mince words about how I feel—not in
a belligerent way, not even as a challenge—love,
wonder, forgiveness—I will say all this plainly so
the words can be heard...not as propaganda, not
as an elder, or as a Christian. To find your life you
must lose it."

You think dogs will not be in heaven?
I tell you they will be there long before
any of us.

Robert Louis Stevenson

*J*ust after my surgery, I noticed that Lulu's chest on the right side had developed a mass—about the size of a child's football. A fatty deposit, I hoped. But it grew larger and Lulu began to slow down. No longer did she lead our beach walks, she lagged behind. And soon she couldn't swim for a stick. She just walked into the water and stood there, grateful for her old ocean friend, as if lost in nostalgia. It was becoming obvious she would not be returning to Maine and our cathedral rock hunts.

I took her to the vet, who did an inconclusive biopsy and put her on antibiotics to bring down a slight fever. I said I suspected she had cancer. When I mentioned my own recent operation, he remarked that it was not unusual for a pet and owner to develop the same disease.

Weeks later X-rays confirmed Lulu's massive breast tumor and another in her abdomen.

Lulu, like other dogs and cats I have known, wanted to die alone and hidden. Twice she ran off into the night after I had let her out to pee.

The first time, when she didn't respond to my constant calls, I worried that she had found a hole or shed to do her dying in, but at 2:00 a.m., suddenly she was standing outside the glass door, too weak to bark or scratch. I let her in with cries of welcome for a friend resurrected.

For a few days she showed signs of recovery, scrabbling into the car for rides to the beach, eating with customary vacuum-cleaner lust. But on the night of a March blizzard, three days before she died, she again ran off into the woods and ignored my calls. After midnight, Annie was shutting off the lights when she spotted Lulu standing in the snow motionless, coated with ice, a white ghost. Again we welcomed her back to our family as if resurrected.

But in the nights ahead she could not sleep, panting constantly and moving from spot to spot every few minutes because of her pain. On March 10, the date my father died, I took Lulu for her last trip to the vet, still uncertain about what to do. The vet said it was time. Lulu didn't notice the injection into her rump. She quietly lay down on a quilt while the doctor, nurse, and I patted her and told her how very loved she was.

The death of my rock hunting buddy hit me like a horrible physical pain. I barely made it out of the vet's office, and on the way home I became a sobbing road menace.

A big saint rock for Lulu.

Franny

DESPAIR IS AN ASPECT OF PRIDE.

St. John of the Cross

{ FRANNY }

I began a new anti-cancer drug, Arimidex. On March 10, Lulu died. On March 14, Holly's 21st birthday.

Annie and I had driven to Hampshire College for a birthday celebration with Holly, recently returned from Barcelona. But I was so exhausted by the drug's effect and depression over Lulu's death, I could barely walk down the street. Life suddenly seemed intolerable. I wanted out.

I called Sloan, told them the drug—or something—was directing me to the exit. I needed help. All my cathedral building, sermonizing and slew of slogans were empty. A simple love of Jesus—gone. Here was suicide and Sloan-Kettering, bless them, knew it. In minutes their suicide team called my motel room: "Have you made plans to kill yourself?" they wanted to know.

Beyond walking out into the freezing night to die, like Lulu wanted, under a bush or in a hole, I had not. That reassured them a bit. I was told to call them back the minute I started making plans.

"You stay here with me Dad. I don't think you should leave. Stay awhile," Holly said, when Annie had to return to Long Island.

I did.

The next week Holly and I visited a local animal shelter. She spotted a black dog huddled in the corner of its cage. "Look at the dog's eyes, Dad. So kind."

We adopted that dog, a border collie mix with energy like a living spark. All thoughts of suicide vanished in that spark

We named her St. Francis of Assisi.

Franny to you.

... I AM MOST IMMODERATELY MARRIED. THE LORD GOD HAS TAKEN MY HEAVINESS AWAY. I HAVE MERGED, LIKE THE BIRD, WITH THE BRIGHT AIR, AND MY THOUGHT FLIES TO THE PLACE BY THE BO-TREE. BEING, NOT DOING, IS MY FIRST JOB.

Theodore Roethke

*H*ope and despair alternated through that summer. About the cathedral I thought little.

When Simon & Schuster's Free Press sent me galley proofs of the hymn book, now titled *Simple Gifts*, I scoffed at my sermonizing there. Hymns were no help now. I considered myself a religious bullshitter and a mere Preacher Boy. For over 60 years I'd had it easy. "You haven't even begun to suffer," I noted in the journal. And I was right. I'd been a privileged word slinger.

I diligently corrected the proofs but my inspiration for the book had vanished.

All churchy chatter and ceremony seemed ridiculous. God talk was just a Scrabble game for career Christians trying to beat the board with fancy words.

Only the Catholic crucifix of the suffering Jesus drew me in. The empty Protestant cross seemed empty indeed. That Catholic guy hanging there knew what it was like.

As for the cathedral—let it crumble into ruins. I busied myself with constructing a 2" x 4" and plank studio for Annie, including electricity for her computer. She would finish a novel there. Before this the camp was an electricity free zone. Now we had a pole and a plug and a utility bill. We were back on the grid.

Pure no longer. But the book Annie wrote, *A Woman of the World*, was later named one of the ten best debut novels of the year by *Publishers Weekly*.

That summer was the 150th anniversary of the Sedgwick Baptist Church—the gold-domed, hilltop symbol of our village. Its stained glass windows are classic and stunning. In the early 19th century it was the Baptist mother church for the peninsula, having converted from its Congregational founding in a switch that was, in that day, sensational. When Sedgwick was a significant port, the church enrolled 400 active members. Now there were four, all elderly. There would probably be no more church anniversaries.

When I walked in the door for that last birthday service I was greeted like a prodigal son. A new member maybe? The start of a re-birth? Pamphlets thrust on me announced that unless I believed, as the surviving four did, that "hell was a real place," I was headed for it.

I fled before coffee hour.

Soon the church was shuttered up and purchased by the Brooklin/Sedgwick Historical Society, who hoped to at least keep its rotting gold dome from crashing into the Benjamin River.

My cathedral was similarly fated. A meaningless discard of rocks. To what purpose? Not even a curiosity.

In July, a close friend of Holly's from high school

days killed herself. Sarah was a vivacious, lovely and funny girl—a Savannah debutante, daughter of a prominent doctor who had prescribed Prozac for her depressions. She wanted to marry a Marine Corps captain and refused to enroll in socially acceptable Randolph Macon College as her parents insisted. When told to break it off with the Marine she put a gun to her head. "Died at home," said the Savannah newspaper obituary cryptically.

For Holly this was the first tragedy of her young life. Unthinkable. She had planned to photograph the wedding for Sarah. They had talked on the phone just days before Sarah shot herself, indicating nothing of her depression, bubbly with excitement.

For Holly and me that summer had to be a recovery of simple faith. There was no way else to go but back to what mattered.

What mattered now was a steel band street dance in the nearby town of Stonington. A Jamaica-inspired assembly of local amateur musicians let loose. Flatlanders and locals cut a rug, as did Holly and I, flailing like flappers in hilarious Sufi joy.

What mattered too was a canoe adventure on the Frost Pond just over the hill from our cathedral site. A bright, windy day on clear, robin's egg blue water—Holly and I paddled into the wind one way and snapped open a red, yellow and orange umbrella for a free ride returning, the wind at our back, laughing.

What mattered was the ancient Kentucky porch swing that Annie had transported to the cabin. On warm days we all took turns napping impossibly deep naps on the swing. In the July afternoons the universe mothered us. For that season at least we were a family with Everything.

What mattered too was sundown cocktails from the tower's peak, the mountains of Acadia visible most days in the haze. Those soft hills had been there for eons and would be long after us.

Curiously, what mattered for me was a huge draft horse at an open house for Blue Hill's Horsepower Farm. A crowd celebrated the machine-free and quite prosperous farm run for generations of the Birdsall family—citizens, children, chickens, pigs, dogs, cats and ambling through it all an unharnessed work horse—an immense, benign, force— the answer it seemed to me to a world of ghastly suffering.

What mattered finally toward the end of that summer was Richard Wyatt, who was driven up to the Pushcart Bookstore by his nurse. Richard is a paraplegic. When he arrived I was correcting *Simple Gifts* galleys on the store's porch out loud. Speaking words is my method of proofing. He was escorted to a chair by his nurse and sat listening for a while.

Later we talked of his Greek Orthodox faith, how a surfing accident and resulting paralysis and constant pain had converted him from a dissolute life to devotion. His physical ruin had become his spiritual birth in the Orthodox Church.

At the end of summer Paul Sullivan told me simply and directly in his studio "Henderson you aren't done yet."

It wasn't a forecast. It was a command.

V
{The Journal}

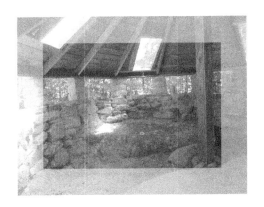

DEATH IS THE RULE TO WHICH LIFE
IS THE EXCEPTION.

Peter Gomes

IT BEGAN IN MYSTERY AND IT WILL
END IN MYSTERY, BUT WHAT A SAVAGE
AND BEAUTIFUL COUNTRY LIES
IN BETWEEN.

Diane Ackerman

{ RIGHT BREAST }

*J*ournal entries recount the next years more precisely and more harshly than I can remember, for indeed many of those days I would like to forget, and have forgotten. A flowing prose would only create a gloss on the deep down horror.

The cancer, it turns out, was not done with me. My stones lay in the woods forgotten. Many days in the years ahead I didn't have the physical strength or the will or the faith to lift them.

Ten million Americans are cancer survivors. Each has their own story of panic, despair and recovery, and many have told these stories in support groups, blogs and books. Each has built a cathedral of hope.

In the next few years I constructed mine, in words and in stone.

10 | 10 | 05

I set 5 symbolic stones at the cathedral—symbolic only. A pledge to return. Days of torrential rain follow, the fall leaves smashed to the ground.

10 | 17 | 05

Two weeks of rain and wind. NW gusts to 50 mph. The Tower shudders beneath me. In the midst of all this a sense that God is watching. I am not alone. Very plain. Like love, it's real. Not to see and feel the Holy Spirit is to live in error.

10 | 19 | 05

I sleep in the Tower. A Harvest moon rises over Acadia's mountains and soothes me in moonlight. It drifts over the sea and trees and at 6 a.m. is still high in the west. The white birches glow in its light. I look for bears gleaning the blueberry fields, but see only moonlight and the beginning of the day... I feel oddly for the first time in a year, blissfully happy.

10 | 19 | 05

Hiking to the Frost Pond, St. Francis of Assisi and I come upon an assembly of birds—two dozen crows on the ground sitting in a circle around an eagle at their center—a mentor, a guru?—in serious discussion. When we crest a hill they exit—the crows in a leisurely flap, the eagle taking his time, a lope into the air where he joins his mate and soars out of sight.

10 | 21 | 05

Back in Long Island, TV again—on Charlie Rose the Dalai Lama says he doesn't need any theology beyond kindness. "I'm just a simple monk. I'd like to make a small contribution."

Later on NBC in Barbara Walters' program

on "Heaven," featuring priests, atheists, Islamic suicide bombers, the Dalai Lama giggles (giggles!) "I'm only a teacher. I just want to be helpful." At program's end, Walters "with the permission of his holiness" kisses his cheek and he in turn enthusiastically rubs noses with her. "Eskimo kiss" he laughs. That's my kind of a god.

11 | 14 | 05

Brother Bob calls—a cathedral saint. For 12 years he's been caring for Debby, his wife. He sleeps on the floor next to Debby's bed, changes her diaper several times a day. The doctors ended her brain cancer (only 5% survive that cancer, they said) but left her helpless, incontinent, paralyzed on her left side. TV is her constant companion. She stares at it endlessly, phoning Bob at his office nearby if she's in trouble. She is his life's work, his total dedication. Her vibrant, wonderful artist's soul has withered, but "she's still in there" he says.

He calls me on his cell phone from a nearby school's running track. Round and round my brother walks in the dark, Debby in the house across the street, her bald head visible in the TV glow. The rolling horror of all this.

11 | 17 | 05

Our father died a stranger to Bob and me. Maybe that's why I choke up so easily at misunderstandings between people. I so wanted to be close to Pop, but his devotion to church doctrines stood between us implacably. He wouldn't discuss his faith.

He left me with a huge hole in my heart.

12 | 6 | 05

Last night the old nightmare, my constant companion. I wander the streets of a strange city. No shoes, ratty clothes. No money. Shunned by all. And no way home.

12 | 8 | 05

Reading again St. Augustine's confessions, my brother from 1,600 years ago. He warns a friend of the addiction of circus violence—the TV drug of the day. Now we have the same vicarious violence but even more gory and explicit than St. Augustine's lions and gladiators. We scarcely blink when entire towns are blown up and Iraqi citizens slaughtered for our evening's TV viewing.

St. Augustine's God is only a spirit to him—forget God's big prick, white beard and sharp sword. Who can pray to that? For St. Augustine, God is love, grace, forgiveness, wonder. That's what you pray to.

Tomorrow mammogram on right breast, my last remaining breast! I'm calm. Expect no surprises. But that may be the problem.

12 | 12 | 05

Mammogram finds spot of calcium near right breast nipple. Deemed "suspicious." Need consultation with Leslie at Sloan-Kettering.

Terror, resignation, fervor for God.

1 | 7 | 06

Saw Leslie Montgomery yesterday at Sloan-Kettering. The old magic still there, a kiss for my girlfriend/surgeon. She pokes me, finds nothing, will ask the radiologist about the film and call me. In any case, not advanced enough to be felt—"Nothing to be alarmed about," says Leslie.

I tell her our two day date at Sloan for removal of my left breast was a joy. "That's because all those lady nurses were taking care of you." Yup. And lovely Leslie in charge.

"Nothing to be alarmed about," walking the ocean beach with the bounding St. Francis of Assisi, I fall on my knees in the afternoon sun. Joy. Gratitude. A resurgence of love for the world. "Nothing to be alarmed about."

GOD IS SIMPLY WHAT ENDURES.

St. Augustine

{LEFT BREAST REDUX}

1 | 20 | 06

The New Year.

Annie and I have rented a house in Sedgwick for the winter—a rehabilitated cottage with windows facing down the Benjamin River. We move in on a warm evening with a full moon.

The phone rings. Leslie. A biopsy is indicated for right breast. "80% of mammograms are negative but still..."

We talk in the bright Maine winter. She's my saint, "A saint rock for you," I say, thank her for saving my life. She's embarrassed by such sentiments, says I am her hero (me, a hero?), not horrified like her other patients. (Women, I think, have a lot more to lose than men from breast cancer.)

So, biopsy it is, in March.

St. Francis of Assisi and I walk up Christy Hill to inspect the cathedral rocks dressed in a light snow.

Would I be strong enough to continue building?

1 | 21 | 06

Phone call. The National Book Critics Circle wants to give me their Ivan Sandrof Lifetime Achievement Award. In New York in March.

Astonishing. Previous winners: Lawrence Ferlinghetti, Elizabeth Hardwick, Alfred Kazin, Pauline Kael, John Updike. I'm dizzy.

Also in March, Poets & Writers says I'm to receive their Writers for Writers/Barnes & Noble Prize. A dinner. A speech.

I can combine biopsy with both.

1 | 23 | 06

Snow! 2 to 3 inches. Plows out—an assault like an army. Snow is war in Sedgwick.

1 | 26 | 06

Surprise, Holly arrives! A snowball's splat on the window announces she's here. She'll be staying all week, working on a documentary film for Hampshire College.

We watch a DVD of "Hearts and Minds," the 1974 film by Peter Davis, who lives nearby in Castine. It's a devastating expose of our war in Vietnam and I've never seen it. I find his number in the phone book and call him. But I'm too moved to speak much. "Thank you" is all I can say. A saint rock for Peter Davis.

2 | 3 | 06

5:15 a.m., 30°, dark—first light coming at 6 a.m. Holly has returned to college. A great sadness. I sit in a dark house. Annie sleeping upstairs. St.

Frances of Assisi on her blanket on the sofa.

Outside on the Benjamin River the amazing force of the tide, a rush as it reaches its fullness under the bridge to Brooklin, almost overtopping it, and then dropping in six hours to leave behind a mud flat. The relentless clockwork power of nature. Last summer young Henry Sullivan and friends swam, laughed and fished from that bridge.

Yesterday at breakfast in Blue Hill with Pastor Rob McCall, he admits "I don't think we will ever really know who Jesus was."

That humility and doubt are what I love about this preacher.

Reading J.D. Crossan's *Jesus: A Revolutionary Biography* "All we are permitted is a glimpse into the mystery..." Jesus was, to Crossan, a Jewish peasant who insisted on the absolute equality of all before God, a healer of the spirit, a wanderer proclaiming the Kingdom of God here and now, a hippie who wanted nothing to do with the trappings of Roman and Jewish authority. For this he was killed and left for the birds to eat. He is resurrected by the love of his followers.

The Roman Empire has left us the smatterings of their lost language and some ruins.

2 | 15 | 06

Paul won a Grammy! He is greeted on his

return from LA by dozens of his young music students at Brooklin Elementary School. They baked chocolate Valentine cupcakes for him and smear him with chocolate joy.

3 | 10 | 06

The biopsy procedure at Sloan-Kettering—face down on a metal table where your male right breast fits into a wide hole. Since I had little to hang there, it was tough for the technicians to milk me like a cow with their extraction tool. I bit my finger hard to cover the pain.

Leslie called days later: "It's cancer!" she announces cheerfully. Why so peppy? I guess because the patient is usually so devastated. Strangely, I'll be glad to see her again. April.

On our trip back from the biopsy and National Book Critics Circle and Poets & Writers awards, Annie and I stop at a Maine Turnpike tollbooth. A wrinkled older woman takes my dollar and I laughingly demand my 15 cents change. She squeezes my hand in affection when handing me the coins. For that small gesture I am moved to tears. Toll takers elsewhere just don't do that. You could lose your toll-taker job. A saint rock for her. Anonymous.

3 | 22 | 06

The local cathedral on this peninsula is the Tradewinds Market, a huge emporium of food, and pharmaceuticals. Plus all your neighbors, and gossip. Here I learn from a neighbor that Maine winters are the brightest of any state in the Union. It's true—sun on snow, sun on the ocean, on the river. It's almost too bright to be depressed.

3 | 23 | 06

A saint rock for Rob Shillady, the one-eyed artist of amazing originality. He paints in his basement while listening to a slew of audio books. Rob and his partner Ellen Booraem, cook Annie and me a terrific dinner—his *coq au vin* specialty. At ice cream time his beeper goes off and so does Rob, slapping a flashing red light on top of his Toyota. Rob is one of two members of the Brooklin first responders. Any disaster, small or large, in any weather, at any time of day or night, and the one-eyed artist is there. Fifteen minutes he's back "False alarm." He spoons up what's left of his melted ice cream.

4 | 16 | 06

Simple Gifts is out. Easter Sunday. Today I sing a hymn on National Public Radio. Free Press booked me on weekend "All Things Considered." Somehow the host of the show convinced me to sing "He Lives" from *Simple Gifts*. "I serve a risen savior, He's in the world today... you ask me how I know he lives? He lives within my heart." A good summary of what I try to believe.

My first national solo, and my last.

4 | 27 | 06

Notes after second breast cancer operation.

The admitting nurse in her warren of an office checks me for vitals—EKG, blood pressure, etc. All surgery patients pass through these offices. "I pray for all of them" she says, and I know she indeed does.

June is her name, a Catholic from Far Rockaway. She lives on the boardwalk in an apartment on the ocean.

She tells me of a horrible accident recently. A beloved young breast cancer doctor, specializing in cancers of young women, was killed outside the hospital by an ambulance driver as she crossed the street. "The sun was in my eyes," he said.

The horror.

Outside June's warren I pass a baby on his way to a PET scan and a beautiful young girl, out cold, on a gurney, coming back from surgery.

At a Slovak Orthodox church down the street I light a candle for all of us, and especially for the person—like young suffering Mark from the first operation—who will be in the bed next to me tomorrow, except turns out, this time I'm alone on the breast cancer ward. All women. I'm quarantined by sex.

Holly and I pledge before the operation to

keep the soul of each other alive. If I die she will keep my spirit and faith alive and I for her. There will be no death for either of us.

Then I walk down the hall in my hospital gown to the room where Leslie awaits me with her team. I lie down on the narrow table and chat with Leslie about Holly and my new book of hymns. I threaten to sing to her. A thing is put over my face. Hours later I'm awake again. "Do you need more pain medicine?" asks the recovery room nurse. I don't.

In my room Holly filches a nurse's latex glove, blows it up. Under a crayoned gap-toothed smiley face she writes "Udderly Happy." The fingers are the udders.

I'm left without udders which I never had anyway, plus tubes running from two drains and memories of my gentle, caring wife and daughter and many nurses.

Leslie is concerned I'll miss my nipples. She suggests they can be tattooed back on. A joke.

Going home the Sloan-Kettering limo driver almost kills us running a red light in Southampton. We are spared a smash up by nanoseconds.

5 | 15 | 06

Rain, rain, rain. Cancer dread. Waiting for the spirit to move across the water to me. Dim visions of the cathedral in Maine, silent in the spring woods.

That spirit arrives in two *Simple Gifts* interviews. The first from Baltimore's WCAO, a black radio station, two guys and me talking about and singing the hymns that join us. No black/white consciousness here. We are one in the old hymns. At closing their "God bless you" is followed by my "God bless you, " words I seldom say, but are real as a hug. I sob.

Hannah Merkel telephones from the Maine *Sunday Telegram*. She tells me her husband died of brain cancer two months before they were set to move to Maine, their dream destination. He loved music, she says, and died listening to Bach's Brandenburg concertos, which she couldn't hear but she could see the solace Bach gave him as he died. She amazingly is deaf. An accident.

She interviews me by assigned phone—she talks and says "Over" and I speak my answer while an operator types my words for her computer. My last words to her typist "God bless you" and I hang up. Sobs, so very deep.

A voice says "Live your book, Bill. They get it right. Why can't you?"

6 | 7 | 06

Back in Maine. Bookstore open. Black flies. Starting the garden.

I learn that early in the 20th century there was a Happy Death movement. And why not, if you aspire to heaven? The best I can imagine of heaven now is an endless, sweet summertime nap on the porch swing.

6 | 10 | 06

Holly's boyfriend's family lives up the road at Stoneset Farm—200 acres of pigs, chickens, goats, sheep, blueberries, vegetables, bee hives and two huge Belgian horses, "Star" and "Julie," 1,700 pounds each. They plough the fields, mud now.

I'm 150 years in the past. Talk at farm dinner is of things of the soil, of new life and slaughter. A pregnant goat stares at me asking what I'm doing there, a stranger from an upscale Hampton resort.

Ginnie, a hospice nurse, and Holly's boyfriend's mom, cares for old Ed. He's 90, losing his sight, the original owner of the farm. Ed joins us for dinner at the picnic tables.

This is what it was like before TV, and radio, when neighbors meant the world to each other, as they still do, at least on this farm.

Around us the first fireflies of the season emerge in the twilight. Above, the full strawberry moon.

6 | 16 | 06

I become a member of the Blue Hill Congregational Church. Rob McCall welcomes me at the pulpit. Since I'm already a Long Island

Presbyterian Elder, I ask Rob if this is theologically legal. He laughs and imagines that it's OK.

7 | 25 | 06

Out of nowhere down the garden path, a riot of flowers, on a sunny spectacular morning appear Charles and Daphine from Lemoine, Georgia. They are seeking the author of *Simple Gifts*. Fans. Baptists. Love the book, passing it out to friends. They hand me $100 for five copies and drive me down the hill in their Lincoln Town car to the Pushcart store to pick them up. On the store porch they ask "Do you believe in the Trinity?"

"I question everything," I answer, "but Jesus, him I don't question."

I don't want them to go, overwhelmed by how much I care about these strangers.

The UPS driver told them where I live, "the tower behind the bushes on the hill."

8 | 4 | 06

6 a.m., gray, drizzle. The rakers have arrived in blueberry fields across the street. For ten hours they will bend to their rakes. French speaking. Haitian, I guess. Two worlds—me on the cabin porch thinking I should get to work on the cathedral when the drizzle stops. Them in the fields, calling out to each other, laughing.

Last night Holly, Annie and I went to hymn

sing at Rockbound Chapel in Brooklin. Holly has a beautiful voice, loves to sing. "His Eye is on the Sparrow" her favorite. Mine too.

The night, bright. Drifting in starlight.

8 | 19 | 06

A candlelight dinner on the cabin porch. Each meal a banquet prepared by Annie.

Annie tells Holly and me about her angel. The angel is real. The angel stays with her, now and then breaking in with a "No!" or "Annie!" as warnings.

Once she was caring for her friend's three year old daughter. The child tottered towards a steep drop. Annie, her back turned, didn't see her. Something flew out of Annie's mouth "NOOO!" The child stopped. Her angel had saved the child's life.

I think perhaps that angel brought Annie and me together.

9 | 1 | 06

Reading Library of America's *Great American Sermons*. Amazing what preachers have spouted in the past. It's almost unrecognizable from the Christianity of today.

I note that Mary Dyer was 13 years old when the New England Puritans hung her for consorting with the devil—the same Puritans who aimed to construct "a shining city on a hill" for all the world to admire—the same "shining city" often cited by politicians as their vision of America.

9 | 5 | 06

Chicken slaughter day at Stoneset Farm. In a 8 x 8' wooden crate dozens of lovely white birds await, straining to see above the rim to understand what's going on. One by one they are picked up and heads stuffed in a cone with necks exposed to be slit. Five bloody cones. Blood on the barn's concrete deck. A bucket of guts. Four ladies, including my friend, sweet Ginny, the hospice nurse, laughing and cutting up bodies fresh from boiling water and defeathering. "Have some chili, Bill! There's a big pot in the house," Ginny sings out.

9 | 6 | 06

At last working on the cathedral again. 60° and gray. No rain. Abandoned idea of a tall edifice. No trebuchet. No hamster wheel. I'm with St. Francis and his humble hut vision. Framing a small door in 2 x 4s, mortaring stone to top the wall all around. Pillars will support the roof and frame the windows—14 of them. A problem. Where to find flat, wild, regular stones for roof pillars? Perhaps Belgian Blocks at the lumber yard? But that's cheating. They aren't wild rocks. The chill is coming. I may indeed cheat.

9 | 12 | 06

Time running out. Cancer checkup next month. 45° in the morning. I order 60 cut granite Belgian Blocks at the Ace Hardware. 3" x 8". $204.56. I cheat.

9 | 18 | 06

Sunday morning. Sun and clouds. 55°. Skip church. Measuring wall for level. Thinking of stained glass windows. But St. Francis would not approve. Mortaring from 9 to 4. It hits 70°—the last 70° for the year probably.

An eagle drifts by, high up, perhaps considering me for lunch.

USA Today article "Three quarters of the US population consider themselves Christian." That translates to 224 million Americans. If Christian, why is this country always at war? Preacher Boy today is of very little faith in "organized" religion.

9 | 22 | 06

55°. I begin to construct the 14 pillars. On top of these pillars I will frame the wooden roof of my St. Francis hut—if the weather holds.

9 | 27 | 06

St. Francis of Assisi and I hike the woods— come upon a 19th century family grave plot—the cellar hole nearby, the house long gone. The tombstones of five children, dead from diphtheria the same year, 1837. Each stone records a testament to faith: "At home with God."

A rebuke to the tepid faith of Preacher Boy.

Dizzy from mixing mortar. Dust inhaled. I'm almost there—14 pillars up, every 22" around the 36' circumference. Room for 13 windows for 13 disciples, including Judas. This by accident.

9 | 28 | 06

52°. At 3 a.m. a porcupine fight in neighbors Jeff and Michelle's apple tree. Hissing and snarling over the apples, they cut off the branches, strip the trees and gobble apples on the ground.

Good news—a tractor trailer filled with hay pulls up. Hay spewed over the blueberry fields for pest control burning later.

Crops next year. No McMansions planned.

9 | 29 | 06

53°. Bought three bags of fine "playground" sand at ACE Hardware for the pew floor.

10 | 1 | 06

I discover what I think is a lump under my left arm. Panic. Depression.

My prayers useless. Am I just a good time prayer?

Letter from a stranger: "*Simple Gifts* touched my heart... your book reminded me of the gift of singing your heart out with thanks, even if the voice is imperfect... I hope your cancer is vanquished... you are a good soul."

10 | 3 | 06

Earthquake last night. 8:10 p.m. Cabin and tower shake maybe 10 seconds. 3.9 on the Richter scale I'm told.

Hundreds of blackbirds swarming south.

10 | 4 | 06

Horrible shooting in Ohio Amish school. A 32 year old man—"a mild man" with kids of his own—invaded a one room school and killed five girls, wounded seven others, killed himself.

The Amish community visited his family in sorrow and forgiveness. Astonishing what a true faith can do.

10 | 9 | 06

Lump definite under left arm. See Leslie 10/19.

At farm dinner Ginny talks of her hospice nursing and how people die. It's a lot easier for those with religious faith. Usually people die gently, their faces relaxed, all tension gone. Sometimes Ginny reminds them "It's OK to stop breathing." And they stop, a tear trickling down a cheek. One man was struggling violently to breathe. She told him to stop. He did.

10 | 11 | 06

Finished St. Francis cathedral rafters, 14 of them connected to the 14 Belgian Block pillars, peaking in a cone.

I am leaving it all for the winter. Lonely cathedral, you still need windows, a door, a roof.

Huge windstorm. The flag is ripped off the tower flagpole.

10 | 20 | 06

At Sloan-Kettering, lovely Leslie finds the lump on her own. "A nugget" she says and biopsies it on the spot with a needle painlessly. "Not particularly alarming," she says.

We talk of her two children, a boy 8, girl 6, and my Holly, and the cathedral, which probably baffles her.

10 | 23 | 06

Leslie calls: cancer in a lymph node. A death sentence I think. It could be any place in my body now.

I crash horribly.

I am a drag on everybody. A cancer sore.

You must know that joy is more rare, more difficult and more beautiful than sadness. Once you make this all important discovery, you must embrace joy as a moral obligation.

André Gide

{A Cross}

10 | 30 | 06

I decide to savor my own death. I look forward to Sloan-Kettering's CAT scan of my entire body and bones and all the cancer to be found there.

But the clicking machines find no new cancer. The admitting nurse did however discover a deer tick dug under my left arm where I couldn't have seen it. Four days of doxycycline due. A tick! How to savor a tick?

But I do learn Preacher Boy has a faith. After Leslie called once again with her cheerful "It's malignant!" I cry out this time not for me, but for all the others with awful diagnoses that hour. I DO care about living and the living. I'd considered blowing my brains out with the shotgun stowed in the cellar, or drowning or freezing or gassing myself rather than continued torture. But when I cried out I found love had not left me. I cried for others.

11 | 10 | 06

Springs. I hit a deer outside the house. Never saw it. The doe lies still in the middle of the road, next to the car's shattered grill. Not breathing. Then it breathes again, struggling with broken legs. I call the police, hear the gun shot. When I return the deer is a heap on the side of the road. Death everywhere.

11 | 11 | 06

How to die? Remembering Pop's quiet death in his sleep after saying his nightly prayers, kneeling at bedside, or Mom in the hospital, gracious, caring, knowing what was coming, "death is no joke" she said—planning to see Pop in heaven soon.

11 | 17 | 06

Surgery. The usual routine.

Leslie finds five bad nodes, more than she expected. Cuts them out. The usual tubes protruding. I spend the night at Sloan, pain free. At 8 a.m., my "vital signs" test, a Jamaican nurse, in her 50's I guess. "How are you?" she asks taking blood pressure. "I'm fine And how are you?" I ask.

"I am having a blessed day," she says. "Every day I wake up is a blessed day."

I choke up. Of course. It's all blessed. She is. Each of us in this cancer hospital is blessed. All the nurses, and doctors and staff. All the patients in their rooms off the main corridors—in their mysterious pain chambers. A teenage girl missing a leg helped by her parents, hobbles down the hall past me as I do laps with my IV apparatus rolling along beside me.

Later, on the beach, St. Francis dashing beside me—"I am blessed. We are all blessed" by the sun and waves and wind, I repeat over and over. That night nurse will never know how her greeting changed one person, taught him again what he knew, and would forget.

12 | 10 | 06

Reading Diana Boss's *Christianity For the Rest of Us.* Why am I reading all these religious books—trying to read my way into faith? The reading of Jesus books may block out the every day Jesus, the sacred moment, and writing may do the same.

12 | 15 | 06

Leslie has ordered chemo, radiation, tamoxifin, in that order. I object. She demands. It's worse that she thought, she says. The Arimidex didn't work. Something has to. We are in trouble here, she says. I have a month to recover from surgery, then we begin with chemo.

St. Francis of Assisi and I travel to Maine—the cathedral needs a roof, at least the peak, because I may no longer be able to reach up that high with my clapboards after treatment.

A week before winter solstice. Gray, cloudy, patches of snow. The garden's brussels sprouts are still edible. I eat them.

12 | 10 | 06

Sunrise far to the south, sinking quickly. When I have gone it will move north again. Again it will climb over Acadia's mountains.

Birthday party last night for 90 year old Charlie Smith. A big gathering of friends and family. His daughter flew in from Scotland. "Old Charlie" sat in a chair and was sung to and lauded in poetry and speeches. Charlie, my regular summer visitor who brought cookies "from the cookie lady" and weed whacked my meadow when I was too weak, and regaled me with WWII recollections of his bombing missions over Germany.

12 | 17 | 06

30°. 7:05. The sun a spark to the south over the sea. Today I begin to clapboard the cathedral roof. Copper and aluminum cone was nailed to the peak yesterday. The clapboard is clear cedar. May last a few years. A stone roof would be better but I'd never sit under a stone roof I erected. Clapboard is light and if it falls on the congregation—me and the dog—we'd be only mildly injured.

From the cathedral's peak, standing on a step ladder in the winter woods, I work down from the copper and aluminum, tedious small cuts to the clapboard as I spread out in a circle that gets wider and wider. I use stainless steel nails that will outlast

the cedar and maybe even the rock walls below. I
want to get the rafters to five feet from the rock
floor. I can reach up that high after radiation and
chemo next summer, I guess.

26°. In the dying light I bang up the last
clapboard.

St Francis and I take a walk to the Frost Pond,
cover the garden with tarps, lock the cabin, tower
and bookstore and at blessed dawn, 16°, leave.

12 | 26 | 06 – Springs

Tests at Sloan—Xrays, CAT, bone and heart
scans, multiple blood drawings.

Holly and I buy a puppy for Annie's Christmas
present, a Portuguese water dog discovered in
a *Newsday* classified ad. All tongue, kisses, and
wiggle for Annie who has endured my illness and
moods with such patience and caring. We name
him Sedgwick.

Where did this cancer come from? The oncologist tosses off "genetics." Six years ago, Holly
had a medical check up before entering Westover
School. They find a breast lump. She's 14. That
night I go berserk remembering my mother and
sister's breast cancer, throwing myself from wall
to wall, Annie horrified. I'd literally lost my mind.
No, No, No! The next day the lump's gone.

Ellen Burstyn, in her marvelous film
"Resurrection," draws diseases from the sufferer

into herself. Impossible? Not in the film. I hope
that's where I got it, a donation from Holly's
young breast. A cure for her.

12 | 30 | 06

Saddam Hussein is hanged. At church I surprise
myself by raising my hand and asking for prayers
of forgiveness for his soul. Forgive? Preaching is so
easy for Preacher Boy.

A local oncologist sticks his fingers in my butt
and proclaims I have "a large, firm prostate without tumor." He wants to put a permanent hole
in my chest, "a port," to deliver chemo for four
months. Miserable, depressed, tired.

1 | 4 | 07

Paul Sullivan calls a happy New Year from
Maine, says he's been praying for me. At the
moment of his call the tide on the Benjamin River
changed, flowing out. He's been watching the river
for decades and never caught it at that moment.
"It means," says my friend, "you're going to be
OK."

1 | 16 | 07

A new oncologist—Susan Emanuel of Twin
Forks Oncology—no life port necessary. Comfy
chairs, choice of musak, I get a haircut since it will
be all on the floor soon anyway.

First infusion. Giant surge in energy from the
steroids. I bloat up, piss a lot. Alternating moods
of hope and what's the use. Don't shave anymore,
no need to.

Is this going to be one of those tough times
producing new insights—or just a tough time lead-
ing to more of the same.

I'm off an island, drifting out to sea in a small
boat. On the island bouncing, chattering, lively
people. I wonder what the racket is about, as I drift
farther, farther away in my boat.

2 | 3 | 07

Bald, lying on the couch in the sun, listening
to Prokofiev's 5th and 7th symphonies, ironic and
frolicking. Chemo slows you down and you actually listen, most days not crammed with energy and
other plans.

Sedgwick doubled in size. He walks with St.
Francis of Assisi (I shuffle) on Sammy's beach every
morning.

2 | 17 | 07

Hannah, my loyal friend and helper with the
Pushcart Prize, had a stroke February 3. Brain
dead. She was 88. Her last act was mailing hundreds of Pushcart Prize nomination announce-
ments written in her beautiful calligraphy. She has
made thousands of writers happy with this news

for 25 years. A great, good and modest woman. A saint stone for her.

I'm raving in anger at Hannah's death.

Chemo and steroids today. Pumped for two days then crash again.

2 | 23 | 07

Wet snow. Trying to think but too exhausted. "Despair is an aspect of pride." OK, but when you are this gone "despair" and "pride" require too much energy to understand. What counts now is the sun suffusing the room, Prokofiev. About cathedrals and the energy that built Chartres I can't even imagine.

Kim is my infusion nurse at Twin Forks oncology. We talk of her dog, Ajax, a five year old German Shepherd and only dog in her husband's Southold Police Canine Unit. Ajax lives with her and their two young daughters and a pug. A beautiful, tender woman.

Hosea Ventura is my PA, a native of the Dominican Republic. Like Kim he is a kind, loving person. These words I still know.

3 | 15 | 07

A tribute to the Pushcart Prize at New York's Baruch College. Joan Murray, editor of the *Pushcart Book of Poetry*, is host. Billy Collins, C.K. Williams, Lucille Clifton, Gerry Stern, Grace

Schulman and Maxine Kumin read. Me, with
fat steroid face and baseball cap over bald dome,
manages a few words of thanks and finds reserves I
didn't know I had.

3 | 21 | 07
    Energy drops to zero. Hanging on to furniture,
just to walk around the house. Where there is no
energy there is no religion.
    Only one word left. Jesus. Banal? No, primitive.
A divinity cared for us. He suffered. He knows. I
can still talk to Jesus, if only from the bottom of
a deep well. After three months of chemo, that's
what's left.

4 | 22 | 07
    Letter from Wendell Berry "I love your book,
Simple Gifts. It is wholehearted, good hearted and
extraordinarily moving—to me and I'm sure to
anybody who treasures the best of old hymns."
Chemo be damned. Wendell lifted me.

5 | 9 | 07
    Lunch with a Pushcart Foundation donor,
Margaret Ahnert, in New York. She's Armenian,
has written a book about the Turkish genocide, lays healing hands on my left arm, says her
Armenian aunt gave her the healing hands and she
passes the healing on to me. We sit in the spring

sun at an outside table at Bistro 60 near Madison
and Park. While crowds hustle by, Margaret sol-
emnly declares I am healed.

5 | 18 | 07

Off chemo, on steroids, ready for radiation.
Thinking—the name of Jesus was all that was
left to me. A fiction, that story. Any attempt to
describe the universe is a fiction, but the real power
is that fiction—the narrative of a suffering, loving
God-man.

5 | 23 | 07

Radiation begins. A four hour daily round trip
drive to Commack, Long Island for 10 minutes
under the giant machine's gun. Left arm over my
head in the mold they made for me.

Horror traffic in and out of the Hamptons.
Surreal. Like an epic DeMille movie. A flood of
pilgrims to the Hamptons. Nuts.

5 | 24 | 07

Holly and eight girls mugged in Baltimore on
their way to a friend's wedding celebration. Two
kids on bikes, a gun—"all cell phones and wallets
on the ground," one kid orders. Holly hands hers
to the kid with the gun. He doesn't shoot her.
Next day she sees him entering a house. Calls cops.
They do nothing.

Holly has not been shot dead. I don't know
what to do with that.

6 | 16 | 07

Last two weeks of radiation. Left chest a
burned steak. Hair returning slowly—a crew cut.
Went to Springs Church, first time in six months.
Old Tom Collins, not seeing me in pew, asks for an
"update on Bill Henderson."

"Tom, I'm here! My hair's back!" I call from
across the sanctuary.

Old militant patriot Tom. WWII vet. American
flag flapping from his SUV antenna. A man whose
politics I could dislike. And it's he who cared about
me, and waves welcome.

Afterwards I tell the new pastor what I had left
deep into chemo was the name of Jesus and the
words "It's not about you."

Pastor Joe says "That about sums it up for me
too."

Bless him.

And suddenly I was back.

7 | 6 | 07

Flee to Maine after last radiation, chest slath-
ered in burn gel.

Holly, staying with her boyfriend, cooks her
first chicken stew for her dad, who is mostly
supine, radiated into near helplessness.

Though the woods I see the St. Francis cathedral, still lacking most of its roof. Two hundred feet away. A long slog it seems now.

I hear radio interview with Norman Mailer.

"How would you like to die?"

"Without undue fear—which is to say with the same confidence I have now that there is another world one enters, and so the finest of all clichés is that death is a great adventure."

I note that. What the minister told my mom as she lay dying. "Dorothy, you are going on a great adventure."

Then, I laughed at the cliché.

Now I don't.

7 | 8 | 07

Garden planted, seed by seed. Bookstore open. Neighbors come by, invite me to dinner. I'm in a mellow malaise, moved by their concern.

Phrase keeps repeating. "It's not about you." As the St. Francis hymn says "Make me a instrument of your peace." Just an instrument.

At Congo church in Blue Hill, Rob opens his sermon with a quote from *Simple Gifts*.

"At the nondenominational Rockbound Chapel, fastened to a granite boulder on a hill over the sea near Sedgwick, Maine, I sing songs with other summer visitors—strangers and people I barely know. In untrained, inelegant, often too-loud or too-soft voices, we sing to each other of our pain, loneliness, and fear, topics we would hesitate to admit flat out in gatherings after services. We also sing of love, grace, trust, hope, peace—sentiments that are left out of the usual daily patter. We sing words that matter to us...

"Our hymns carry all of us to those Thin Places described by the Irish, elevated states of consciousness where almost all barriers between mortals and gods vanish..."

8 | 3 | 07

We dine on Annie's fine cuisine on the cabin porch as a big orange moon rises over the distant sea. The night is cool and bright and the wine flows and peace descends on our little family.

Just before dawn a coyote convention nearby. Everybody voting. A howling clatter. I bring St. Francis and Sedgwick inside. Coyotes and dogs are not friends.

8 | 16 | 07

The first morning glories bloom. Two hummingbirds arrive to drink from the soft blue celebrations.

The garden is lush—kale, summer squash, pole beans, tomatoes—all rushing to beat the dying of the sun.

I'm stunned by summertime grace.

8 | 30 | 07

Doris Grumach and Sybil Pike rent a house on a cove nearby. Doris and I talk sitting in the sun. Doris says she attends Ash Wednesday services, but she has no use for Easter. "The resurrection is a myth of the church…On the cross, that's where I leave him."

I tell Doris what the name Jesus meant to me during chemo and how the phrase "It's not about you," freed me.

"It's like you realized possibility again," she says.

Indeed I was free from my own tired proclamations, my own husk.

When Doris had a terrible attack of shingles years ago, the intractable pain drove her to thoughts of drowning herself in the cold ocean.

Doris on writing: "In old age we should throw away our notes and just write from the heart."

9 | 3 | 07

Much media blather about Mother Teresa and her dark night of the soul. Just revealed in her letters and journals. "In my soul I feel that terrible pain of loss," she wrote in 1959. "Of God not wanting me—of God not being God—of God not existing." The agony lasted until her death in 1997.

She recalls that Christ suffered the same sense of abandonment by God on the cross and that the

Calcutta poor she helped were always abandoned.
Atheists rejoiced—called her a fraud saint.
These atheists imagine that faith is too easy and
believers too simple. As Rob McCall admits, sometimes faith evaporates, but for him and for many
of us, it returns. Besides, as I noted, I don't know
enough about God to be an atheist.

9 | 4 | 07
Clear, clean air. Thinking of when I first drove
up the dirt road to Christy Hill years ago. The
sense of unlimited time (the mountains of Acadia),
space (I imagine you can see the curve of the earth
from the tower top). Call it God, if you will. Here
I am submerged in the holy, always every day, if
I'll just pay attention. No more mottos about what
should be. Here I am a sponge for the Great Spirit.

9 | 5 | 07
Fashioning plexiglas skylights for the cathedral,
to be nailed to the roof frame—North, South,
East, West. This will not be a gloomy sanctuary.
Light everywhere. St. Francis would approve of the
light. My ideas of rock permanence not so much.

9 | 10 | 07
Holly calls from New York. She ran in the 3K
Susan G. Komen Breast Cancer Run in Central
Park. 20,000 runners. On her back a sign "In

memory of my grandmother. Thanks for survivors, my aunt and my dad."

9 | 11 | 07

Pole beans ready! Just picked! Steamed! Heaven!

On the way to Congo church in Blue Hill I see neighbor Parker Waite on the road. Stop.

"Going to church?" I ask.

"I don't believe any of it," he laughs.

"It's all in your heart—God is there."

"My heart is nasty and mean."

"No it's not Parker. You are a very kind person. That's where God is."

"He doesn't exist," snorts Parker.

And I drive off alone, conversion attempt having failed. I will try again.

9 | 21 | 07

The last warm days. I set a large flattish stone at the cathedral doorway and continue with clapboards moving down the roof side.

9 | 22 | 07

I fashion a cathedral door from pine planks, varnished and hinged. This is a small door. It is low. You must bend way down to enter this cathedral. If you don't you will bang your head.

Rob McCall says that's a Navajo concept—the

kiva. You go down to enter a round sacred circle. Who knew?

9 | 23 | 07

I finish the roof at 5:46 p.m. today, Sunday. Needs a bit of trim, but the cathedral is now complete, the broken-hearted, sacred rock covered with a #1 red cedar clapboard roof—something new for it after millions of years.

In one of the windows, a seaside one, I hang a cross Doris gave me—part of a destroyed lobster trap we guess, two waterlogged sticks connected by a single rusty nail, washed up on the beach rocks. I hang it from a rafter. Otherwise the dome is empty of artifice.

As the early fall light fails, I sit on the sacred rock and remember my first congregant—Lulu— my arm around her. Lulu and I sit empty-minded again, silent, watching the sea. Dog, human. Wordless in the mystery.

{ABOUT THE AUTHOR}

BILL HENDERSON IS THE FOUNDING EDITOR of the Pushcart Prize series. He received the Ivan Sandrof Lifetime Achievement Award from the National Book Critics Circle and the Poets & Writers / Barnes & Noble Writers for Writers Award.